Lesley Ackland with Eva Gizowska

15-Minute Pilates

Body Maintenance to Make You Longer, Leaner and Stronger

Thorsons
An Imprint of HarperCollins*Publishers*

Thorsons

An Imprint of HarperCollins*Publishers*

77–85 Fulham Palace Road,

Hammersmith, London W6 8JB

First published 1998

10 9 8 7 6 5 4 3 2 1

A catalogue record for this book
is available from the British Library

ISBN 0 7225 3776 X

↝

Text illustrations by Peter Cox

Printed and bound in Great Britain by
Woolnough Bookbinding Limited, Irthlingborough, Northamptonshire

15-Minute Pilates

Lesley and I both have Pilates-based exercise studios. We both agree that the individual is more important than the technique. Lesley trained with me and the focus of both our studios and teaching approach is based on each client's individual and very specific requirements.

Alan Herdman
Pilates' pioneer in the UK

Contents

Preface

HOW TO USE THIS BOOK

Do you dream of a flat stomach, a longer, leaner body and superb posture?
Do you wish to improve your overall appearance? If so, then *15-Minute
Pilates* will help you achieve all this – and more. In this book you will
discover a unique bodywork system that will help you transform your body
and develop a physical presence and energy that exudes total confidence
and grace. If you want to become healthier, stronger, leaner and more
supple, my Pilates-based Body Maintenance techniques are designed to
work for *all* ages and *all* levels of fitness. There are also specific remedial
techniques you can try if you suffer from medical conditions such as a bad
back, scoliosis, repetitive strain injury (carpal tunnel syndrome) or sciatica.

While most people have heard of Pilates, few know exactly what it entails.
Pilates is a very disciplined, focused form of exercise, designed to strengthen
ligaments and joints, increase flexibility and lengthen the muscles. The
main emphasis is on 'elongating' the body to create a longer, leaner and
taller silhouette. However, Pilates differs from other exercise regimes by
going beyond the purely physical. This is a holistic discipline that integrates
the mind, body and spirit. It is a philosophy of movement that brings about
mental and physical integration.

If you have never tried this type of exercise before, you will be surprised by its apparent simplicity. The slow, controlled movements enable energy to move more freely throughout the body. The visualization techniques gently help to focus the mind so that each exercise is executed with ultimate precision. With Pilates there is no need for over-exertion. The emphasis is on *quality*, not quantity. It's not about how much you do but, rather, how you do it. This is good news indeed for those of you who have become disillusioned and bored with fitness programmes which may not suit you.

If you want to have a long, lean look, with a minimum of effort in the safest way, you merely have to follow the guidelines in this book. Most of the techniques are based on the idea of using your own body to create resistance, so there is no need for any complicated props. All you need is a willing body and a curious mind. Before you attempt any of the exercises though, it is important that you first become acquainted with the underlying principles.

In the Introduction I outline the profound effect Pilates has had on my own life, and how I have evolved and updated this classic regime to make it more contemporary and accessible. Chapter 2 explains how my Pilates-based Body Maintenance Programme works, and what you can hope to achieve. It explains how much easier it is to bring about physical changes when you learn to focus your mind and practise visualization techniques as well.

Chapter 3 covers the basic principles of Pilates, such as the importance of proper breathing, stretching, posture and movement control. It introduces the key terms which are used throughout the book, and explains the physiological effects of Pilates techniques on your body. For practical advice on clothes, safety, equipment and which exercises you should do, turn to Chapter 4.

The core exercise programme is outlined in Chapter 5. Here, you will find a 'menu' of all the different types of exercise you can do, for 15 minutes, at home, every day. They include exercises to tone and strengthen your abdominal muscles, the muscles in your back, your upper body (arms, chest and shoulders) and your lower body (legs, hips and thighs), as well as a series of all the essential stretches.

If you suffer from any of the following – a bad back, scoliosis, repetitive strain injury (carpal tunnel syndrome) or sciatica – then you will find the relevant remedial exercises signposted in Chapter 6. Finally, in Chapter 7 you will find some case studies of people who have benefited from my Pilates regime.

15-Minute Pilates is no idle promise – that's all it takes, a quarter of an hour every day, to see results. Too good to be true? Why not see for yourself? You will be pleasantly surprised.

Acknowledgements

I dedicate this book to Thomas Paton and Brenda Eliel for their support and encouragement.

A big thank you to all my clients, and Nick Ringham, Jo Lynn and Andrew Jost.

For further information on The Body Maintenance Studio please send a stamped addressed envelope to:

Body Maintenance Studio
2nd Floor
Pineapple
7 Langley Street
London WC2H 9JA

1

Introduction

With Pilates I believe that you can achieve the body you want in a controlled, progressive and intelligent way. It can give you the shape you want. Pilates doesn't build bulk, but strengthens weak muscles and stretches tight ones. You can concentrate on one part of the body without straining another. Pilates differs from other forms of exercise as it initially focuses on posture. Good posture is essential in realigning the body, which can have you looking and feeling taller, slimmer and well-toned.

The beauty of Pilates is that it is suitable for people of all ages. Notwithstanding your level of fitness, you have the potential of achieving a supple body and reaching a level of 'wellness' that you will want to maintain. You should feel good about yourself, which involves an intelligent dialogue between your body and mind. Imagery and visualization are very appropriate tools – if you can focus on how you wish to look, the body will most assuredly co-operate. How you picture yourself is reflected in your body language which, in turn, is observed by the world at large. When that language is fluent and flowing you will be aware of it – others will comment on how well you look.

For those who have repetitive strain injury (carpal tunnel syndrome), scoliosis or a myriad of other problems, Pilates is a superb tool to use as you begin the journey towards helping and even reversing your condition. I believe that everyone can and will improve and even overcome their physical liabilities, with a safe and gentle group of exercises. You will be amazed at the body's ability to respond and rejuvenate given the correct impetus. For those of you with serious postural problems involving balance, Pilates can change not only your body, but the perception of vulnerablity you feel and transmit to others. You will regain your confidence and not live in fear of falling, stumbling and giving the impression of vulnerability to others who could cause you injury.

I have never met anyone I could not help with Pilates. We should not tolerate a life which is limited due to 'the back', 'the leg', etc. To embrace such negative thinking is to resign oneself to a very unsatisfactory existence and lifestyle. As you begin the following exercises be patient but determined, and feel the body working towards what you have always envisioned – the elegance of a swan's neck, the supple back of a ballet dancer. Feel yourself floating – soaring as you go through your movements. Concentrate on the moment, eventually all will be remembered as you progress. Even those of you who are extremely unfit can look forward to the day you can look in the mirror and not recognize your former selves.

THE PILATES' EFFECT

Until quite recently, the majority of people who knew of Pilates were dancers. It was a relatively unknown technique that had been brought to England by Alan Herdman. The beauty of Pilates is that it engages the body and mind simultaneously. The actions, which are gentle and flowing, promote excellent tone, sleekness and grace. This was exactly what I was looking for, and I quickly realized this method could revolutionize the way in which people exercise.

As my interest in Pilates grew, I was ready for a career change. Even though I had an excellent job as head of business studies at a large school in North London, I felt ready to move on. I decided to leave teaching and trained with Alan Herdman. I studied remedial physiotherapy as well, then furthered my Pilates' study in New York. For five years I was the Remedial Exercise Consultant to the Birmingham Royal Ballet.

The Body Maintenance Programme that I teach today is a Pilates-based regime with a modern twist. It combines classic Pilates with a variety of new techniques which have evolved along the way, to suit people of all ages and levels of fitness. I like to call it the thinking person's exercise, because it is very creative and it inspires the mind to re-shape the body. The fact that you have to think and analyse what you are doing precludes boredom. Once you have mastered some of the techniques in this book, you will see for yourself how totally absorbing and exciting it is.

THE ORIGINS OF CLASSIC PILATES

The original concept of Pilates was the brainchild of a German, Joseph Hubertus Pilates. He was extremely frail and weak as a child, but was determined to regain good health. This was the start of a life-long obsession with fitness and body building, and as a young man he excelled as a diver, skier and professional gymnast. Aged 32 he decided to move to England, where he made a living as a boxer, circus performer and self-defence instructor.

When the First World War broke out, his career was temporarily cut short. As a German, Pilates was interned in England for the duration of the war. He used this time, however, as an opportunity to re-think and develop his approach to fitness. The result was the first blueprint for a whole new regime, Pilates, which drew upon all the various disciplines with which he was involved. His basic philosophy concluded that the only way to achieve true fitness was through the integration of mind and body. Hence, all his techniques were based on a combination of physical and mental conditioning.

When Joseph Pilates created his unique system of exercise during the early part of the twentieth century, the lifestyle was, in many respects, healthier for the public at large. Without the profusion of cars and mass transportation, walking was not merely a preferred form of exercise but, rather, the efficient way of getting from place to place.

Many of the injuries and disabilities of the 1990s are, in fact, caused by our very modern, machine-oriented society. Repetitive movements on computers and sitting in an office chair for the greater part of the day contradicts the physiological needs of the human body. There are, of course, factors beyond our control, such as genetic traits and unfortunate injuries, which must also be addressed. I knew that I had to expand and enhance the basic principles of Pilates.

BODY MAINTENANCE – A NATURAL PROGRESSION

The aim of my Pilates-based Body Maintenance Programme is to pin-point what is causing a particular imbalance to occur in the first place. I tend to view it as a problem solving exercise. First, I look for the root of the problem, then I try to provide a solution through specific exercises. Body Maintenance is all about asking the right questions. My clients initially wish to address specific problems with the presupposition that their manifestations of pain or discomfort stem from only one region of the body – the area in which the pain is most acute. More often than not, after observing their movements, obtaining relevant medical histories and getting a sense of their lifestyles, they are thoroughly surprised when I explain that the actual source of their discomfort is not, in fact, limited to 'the neck' or 'the hip', but rather has a variety of causes which may have arisen long before the sign became a symptom.

I try to assess not only the physical problems but the feelings that accompany them. Physical distress has a huge impact on the emotions. Using my Pilates-based methods, I then design a personalized exercise routine suited to each client. Pilates recognizes that whatever the problem, no two situations are exactly alike. As a result, I believe that both the physiological and psychological factors must be taken into account. Thus, the mind–body connection. The successful execution of a simple exercise

5

depends as much on the cerebral willingness as on the physical abilities. I am constantly changing, altering and making up exercises all the time. I have customized some of the moves so that now someone can come into my studio and do an hour-and-a-half of foot exercises, for example.

For those of you who wish to enhance or change some aspect of your bodies, this routine is simple and straightforward. People tend to use their big muscles for everything. I work on strengthening the smaller muscles – the obliques – which can give you the shape that you want. You can tone your stomach, thighs and arms and reshape your buttocks as well. Get into swimsuit shape – look and feel longer, leaner and more glamorous. Stomach muscles have an unusually short memory. Daily reminders will keep them taut and toned. There is no limit to what you can expect to achieve. My workout will have you feeling supple, slender and self-assured. Your entire view of yourself, both physically and emotionally, will improve and you will reach that summit of 'wellness' where the mind–body–spirit positively connect. The rest is up to you.

2

The
Theory

THE MIND–BODY CONNECTION

The main principle of Pilates is that exercise is essentially a mind–body technique. Therefore, when you exercise you mentally focus on the muscle groups that you are using. Pilates recognizes that it is only through the synchronizing of thought and action that an exercise is truly effective. In order to create a healthy and fit body you need to integrate the mental, physical and spiritual spheres.

MIND OVER MATTER

It has long been established that the mind has a enormous influence on the health of the body. Research shows that the mind has an infinite capacity to induce positive physiological effects, which have both an internal and external effect. You may have noticed that when you're in a good mood you automatically seem to look and feel better. Scientists ascribe this phenomenon to the activity of the billions of nerve cells in our brain, which transmit chemical messages to the rest of the body. Our thoughts and emotions play a vital role in influencing this intercellular communication.

Think for a moment how you feel when you are stressed. Not very pleasant. This is because your body produces an excess of 'stress' chemicals (e.g., adrenaline and cortisol), which causes your whole system to speed up. Your heart beats faster, your blood pressure goes up, your breathing becomes rapid and shallow. At times, this type of response is necessary. It is what motivates you when you are faced with a crisis. In large doses this type of reaction can, however, be extremely harmful and can lead to all sorts of unpleasant symptoms such as dizziness, shaking, profuse sweating, insomnia and migraines. It is easy to see what effect negative, stress-inducing emotions can have.

Positive feelings of calm and contentment have a much more beneficial effect, as they induce the body to produce health enhancing, feel-good chemicals (e.g., endorphins and serotonin), which are vital for well-being. They promote a sense of serenity – you breathe more easily and deeply, your heart rate is slower and your blood pressure lowers. The more relaxed you feel, the less tension you hold in the muscles throughout your body. This has a beneficial effect on your general bearing and posture. Tight, tense muscles make your body shrink and constrict. This stops the energy from flowing freely throughout the body and, in time, this will be reflected in a weak, misshapen musculature.

MINDFUL EXERCISE

If thoughts are so powerful, it makes sense to try and harness your thinking to bring about positive changes in your body. This is, in fact, the very essence of Pilates. By learning to execute each exercise correctly you are also allowing your mind to exert a greater influence over your body. With Pilates you only do a limited number of repetitions. You do them slowly, so that you can concentrate more clearly on directing your energy towards what it is you are trying to achieve. If you view your body in a negative way you will need to reverse your direction of thought. Positive thoughts bring about positive changes.

9

To ensure that an exercise can be of real benefit and bring about the changes that you desire, for example a strong, straight back, it is necessary to complement each physical action with a mental focus. By practising creative visualization regularly, you will gradually develop the intellectual and emotional ability to internalize the physical changes that you wish to make. Once you've done this, the external changes will start to appear.

The Theory

As you become aware of your body and its needs, you can consciously start to make changes through exercise. Pilates is based on lengthening and stretching the body to its full potential. This eventually creates a longer, leaner shape, increased flexibility and a suppleness that promotes a greater ease of movement. These exercises concentrate on strengthening weak muscles and stretching those which are too tight and constricted. What you really want is a body in which strength and flexibility complement each other. It is possible to totally re-structure the way you are. It is not, however, just a matter of getting your body to make the right moves. An integral part of Pilates is the way you perceive the exercise. This is why attitude and creative imagery are so important. Each time you work through a series of movements it is essential that you can envision what it is that you wish to achieve. Painting a picture in your mind helps your body to respond in the right way. This not only makes the whole process more stimulating but the effects of each exercise are much more powerful. Initially it may take a while to fully understand the mechanisms. I always tell a new client to expect to do only about 30 per cent of what he or she will eventually be capable of doing. It takes about 10 sessions to really comprehend the technique. Pilates is the only form of exercise that gets progressively more difficult, but the results are worth it. In time you will look taller, slimmer and more toned.

CREATIVE VISUALIZATION

Whatever we create in our lives begins as a basic image in our minds. Many of these images are unconscious. Through creative visualization it is possible to alter these thoughts and pictures. With Pilates, the idea is to create an image in your mind that will help you to focus on the area of the body that you are working. This requires a very deep level of concentration, which does become easier with practice. On a superficial level, many of the exercises appear quite simple. How you physically position your arms and legs, however, is only part of the process. Pilates, unlike many other disciplines, is actually much more complex as with each movement you must be constantly aware of what your entire body is doing. You don't concentrate only on the stomach, or the inner thigh, and exclude the rest of your body. Even when you are doing a series of movements specifically designed to work a certain group of muscles, such as your abdominals or your quads, you must always remember to be equally focused on the rest of your body. Where are your feet? Are you holding your head in exactly the right way? Is your body properly aligned?

Initially, this can seem quite difficult and using visualization techniques can be enormously helpful. By understanding how your body should be feeling it becomes easier to assume the correct position. Eventually, these images will arise naturally through association, without too much effort. Visualization is one of the best methods to bridge the gap between mind and body. By creating mental pictures that correspond to what you are trying to do physically you will, in time, develop a level of body awareness which is unique to Pilates.

Basic Techniques

Anyone can learn to visualize. It helps though if you can begin by feeling relaxed. A still mind is more conducive to conjuring up images.

- *Spend a few minutes gathering your thoughts. Try to forget about external influences such as work, what you should be doing and any worries you might have. Remember, this is your time.*
- *Do some gentle stretches and focus on your breathing. Slow, deep breathing has an instantly calming effect because it helps to promote soothing alpha brainwaves. Once you are feeling sufficiently relaxed you can start your exercises.*

- *As you exercise, focus on each part of your body. How does it feel? With each exercise try to perceive a specific picture. If you are trying to envision yourself on a sandy beach, focus clearly on how this feels. Do your feet feel relaxed, warm and comfortable? Are your arms hanging loosely by your sides, like a puppet? Where is your head? Think of images that will help you to get into exactly the right position.*
- *Invite each image to emerge with as much intensity as possible, so that you can almost feel it. Once you have created a familiar picture, eventually all you will have to do is to focus on it and your body will automatically respond.*

The concept of Pilates is to bring about permanent changes. You can hasten this process by using visualization techniques when you are not exercising. These will automatically help you to walk, stand and sit in the correct way.

THE GOLDEN RULES

Pilates-based Body Maintenance is a very precise system of exercise. It is different from other regimes in that it requires a bit of groundwork before you start. In order to understand fully what you are doing it is important that you first become acquainted with the basic principles. There are six essential guidelines to remember.

1. Concentration

Rather than perceiving exercise as a mindless activity, it helps if you can develop a focused approach. This not only makes the whole process more stimulating, but also ensures that you are exercising correctly. Maintaining concentration is possibly the most important aspect of Pilates. The exercises are so subtle as to appear simple, but the reality is that every movement requires total concentration. Initially it takes time and commitment to ensure that you are focusing on doing each exercise in precisely the right way. It's not just a case of adopting a position and working through the movements. It is vital that you are aware of the rest of your body throughout. This may seem rather demanding at first. With each exercise, you not only have to remember how to position your arms and legs, but you must master all the rules of correct alignment as well. Furthermore, you must focus on the muscle or group of muscles you are working. This is where visualization can really be helpful. You can use this technique to recall how every sensation should feel. Once you have learned the art of total focus, you will no longer be able to conceive of exercising any other way.

2. Control

Concentration will help you to control your every movement and every breath. With Pilates every move counts – from how you hold your head to where you place your fingers. It takes a while to reverse the poor habits of a lifetime of not being aware of body alignment. We slump in our chairs, hunch in our cars and then wonder why we're not as supple and flexible as we could be! Pilates is all about coaxing the body into proper alignment. You should be aware of what your body is doing at all times. It is only by making a conscious decision to transform your shape that unconscious changes can take place.

3. Centring

The main principle of the Pilates technique is to recognize that there is one strong, core area that controls the rest of the body. This is located in that part of your body which forms a continuous band at the back and front,

The Theory

between the bottom of your rib-cage and across the line of your hipbones. This is called the *centre*. This is the area in which the muscles in your stomach and back are – at the centre of your body. These muscles support the internal organs and keep you upright. If you have a strong centre you have a strong back, which means you can walk, stand and run without discomfort or pain. Your arms and legs are extensions of this part of your body. If you have a bad back this is an indication that the centre is not strong enough. Originally human beings were not designed to stand upright. The only reason we stand at all is due to these specific muscles. We are constantly fighting gravity, which pulls us forward. This explains why so many people have all sorts of problems with those muscles affiliated with the shoulders and neck. We are basically defying nature, gravity and our initial body type.

4. Flow

Each movement in Pilates is designed to be performed in a smooth, flowing, undulating way. There is no room within this regime for any sharp, jarring movements or quick, jerky actions – these are the total antithesis of everything you are trying to achieve. If a movement ever feels like this, you can be sure you are doing it wrong. Every motion originates from a strong centre and flows in a slow, gentle, controlled fashion, thus warming the muscles and causing them to lengthen and open up the spaces between each vertebra in the spine so that the body expands to create a longer, leaner shape.

5. Precision

In order to be effective, all Pilates exercises have to be performed with exact precision. This attention to detail is important as it ensures that each movement is working the body in the correct manner. Before you start an exercise sequence, read the instructions carefully. Pay full attention to proper alignment and check what the 'watchpoints' have to say. This will ensure that you do not expend excess energy when an exercise is not done correctly.

6. Breathing

The importance of breathing is covered in the core exercise programme. The main thing to remember is to follow all the breathing instructions which accompany each exercise.

The Body

Before you begin the Pilates programme, try this simple preliminary body awareness exercise.

Standing or sitting, close your eyes. Take a few deep breaths and, starting with your head, slowly direct your focus down through your entire body. Imagine that you are steering the flow of energy throughout your body. As you do this try to visualize all the different parts of your body along the way. Think of your eyes, ears, mouth, down the shoulders, arms and hands. Visualize your chest, back, abdomen, hips, pelvic area, upper legs, knees, lower legs, ankles and feet. As you visit each area try to build up a mental picture of how it looks and feels. Spend a few seconds tuning into each part. Move your head gently, shrug your shoulders. Gently move your stomach, tailbone and hips. As you do this, concentrate on the sensation. Which areas feel most comfortable and relaxed? Are certain areas tight and constricted? Do this for a few minutes each day. This will help you to become more aware of your body when you are ready to begin the exercises.

KEY TERMS

In Pilates there are certain key terms that are referred to over and over again. It helps if you understand these before you begin.

Relaxing

Pilates frequently refers to keeping an area *relaxed*. This isn't necessarily what you might think. Most people associate relaxation with a feeling of 'letting go', of allowing muscles to slump. In this case, to relax means to release tension in an area while still managing to maintain tone and control. This should feel comfortable and natural.

Neutral Spine

Some of the positions you will be assuming require your spine to remain in *neutral*. This means that you maintain the natural curve in your back. Thus, when you are lying down, do not press your back so hard into the floor that you lose your natural curve. Neither must you allow your back to arch so that your lower back comes off the floor. Just lie there, breathe in and out naturally and allow your back to relax into the floor without pressing it in. This will permit your back to relax into its natural, neutral position – which is slightly different for everybody.

The Centre

With Pilates, every exercise originates from the *centre*. The stomach muscles are the core to everything and support the spine. It is important that you always remember to keep this area correctly aligned. This is particularly important when you exercise the lower abdominals as it is very easy to do the opposite of what you actually want. It is natural when you breathe in for the stomach to pull into the spine and when you breathe out for it to bulge. This is not what you want. You will have to try and reverse what the body wants to do unconsciously. As you breathe in you should relax the stomach; as you breathe out you should pull the navel to the spine, engaging the lower abdominal muscles. Your body will naturally want to do the opposite, but it's important to engage the stomach muscles when you exhale.

The Body

The Feet

The main thing to remember when exercising is that most of the time you want your feet to be relaxed. If you are in doubt – relax your feet. Most people tense their feet too much and as a result constantly complain about getting cramp in their feet when they are exercising. (If you do get cramp use a foot roller to ease away the tension.) A relaxed foot should feel comfortable, so that there is no sensation of tightness. Whenever you are required to flex your feet, do so by gently stretching out your heel then pulling the top of your foot as far as you can without straining. Do not tense your foot so that it feels strained.

The Neck

This is a sensitive part of the body, so you do not want to put it under unnecessary strain while you are exercising. It is very important that you always follow the neck instructions very carefully. Pilates often refers to *keeping your neck long*, which means adjusting your head into a position that lengthens your neck. When you are doing an exercise lying on your back, the way you bring your head into alignment with the rest of your body is by moving the top of your skull and the base of your neck. Do not attempt to flatten your neck against the floor.

Straight Arms and Legs

This is a very common term in Pilates. Your arms and legs should be relaxed and not locked. This is an important point to remember, particularly for the stretches. If an exercise requires that you stretch your arm or leg out straight, you should take care not to overextend, causing the joints to lock.

BODY BASICS

The main function of the skeletal system is to provide your body with support, protection and movement. Bones act as levers and when muscles pull on the bones, this causes parts of the body to move. Muscles are attached to the bones by tendons comprised of tough, fibrous, non-elastic connective tissue. The bones you should be most concerned about in Pilates are the main 25 bones that comprise the spinal column, consisting of:

- *seven cervical vertebrae in the neck*
- *twelve thoracic vertebrae articulating with the ribs in the thorax*
- *five lumbar vertebrae in the lower back*
- *four bones fused together into the coccyx at the base of the spine.*

One Vertebra at a Time

Pilates frequently refers to the term *one vertebra at a time*. This is one of the main principles that you should keep in mind whenever you are doing an exercise that involves rolling your body up from and down to the mat. The idea is that you always roll up gradually so that you are lifting only one vertebra off the mat at a time. The same rule applies when you roll back down again. This takes some practice and initially you will need to concentrate very carefully to ensure that you are doing it correctly.

Movements

All movements involving the bones occur at the joints, thus enabling a variety of different movements. The more common ones that you are likely to come across in Pilates include:

The Body

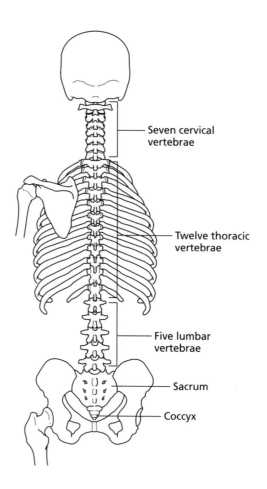

Seven cervical
vertebrae

Twelve thoracic
vertebrae

Five lumbar
vertebrae

Sacrum

Coccyx

Flexion – *which bends a limb or the spine, e.g. when bending the head forward onto the chest.*

Extension – *which straightens a limb or the spine.*

Hyperextension – *which means bending back further than the vertical position, e.g. moving the head backwards to look up at the ceiling.*

Abduction – *when you make a move away from the centre of the body, e.g. raising your arms horizontally sideways.*

Adduction – *when you move towards the centre of the body, e.g. you lower your arms to the sides.*

Inversion – *when something turns inwards, e.g. you turn the sole of your foot inwards.*

Rotation – *when the bone turns on its axis either away from or towards the centre of the body.*

The Muscles

Muscles create a movement by exerting a pull on the tendons which move the bones at the joints. They are also responsible for maintaining posture. Many muscles are attached by the tendons to two articulating bones. Most movements, therefore, involve the use of several muscle groups. Muscles may also work in 'antagonistic' pairs – one muscle contracts to move the bone in one direction; the other muscle contracts to move it back, e.g. the calf and shin muscles which raise and lower the foot. Each muscle has the ability to contract or shorten. It can be stretched when it is relaxed. Muscles also control internal functions such as pumping blood round the body and the propulsion of food through the digestive system. There are literally hundreds of muscles in the body (there are 620 muscles which can be consciously controlled alone), all of which are involved in a wide range of functions.

The most important muscles you should be aware of for the purposes of Pilates are:

The Body

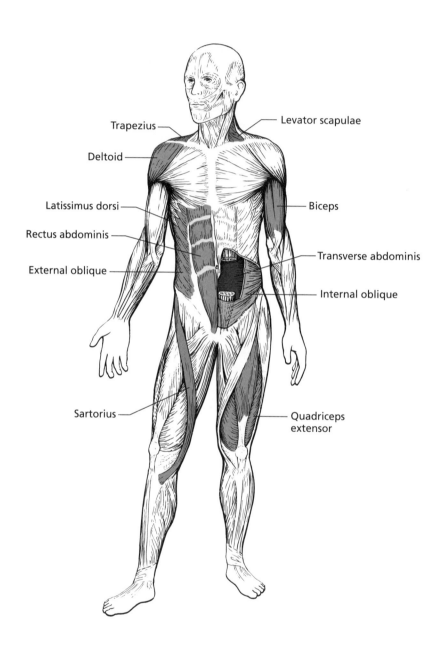

Trapezius

Levator scapulae

Deltoid

Latissimus dorsi

Biceps

Rectus abdominis

Transverse abdominis

External oblique

Internal oblique

Sartorius

Quadriceps extensor

15-Minute Pilates

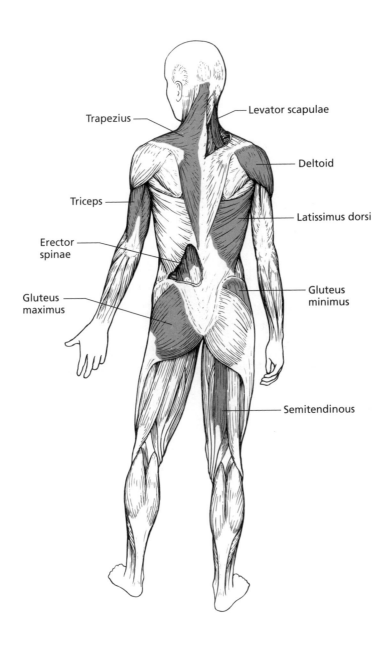

Trapezius

Levator scapulae

Deltoid

Triceps

Latissimus dorsi

Erector
spinae

Gluteus
minimus

Gluteus
maximus

Semitendinous

The Body

Trapezius – *in the back of the neck running down to the shoulders.*

Action – *extends the head.*

Levator scapulae – *at the back and sides of the neck, running into the shoulder.*

Action – *lifts the shoulder blade and shoulder.*

Deltoid – *on top of the shoulders and upper arms.*

Action – *moves the arm backwards and forwards.*

Biceps – *at the front of the arms.*

Action – *moves the arm.*

Triceps – *at the back of the arm.*

Action – *moves the arm.*

Gluteus maximus – *form the buttocks.*

Action – *raises the body, used in running and jumping.*

Gluteus minimus – *in the buttocks.*

Action – *rotates thigh laterally, maintains balance, used in walking and running.*

Sartorius – *crosses front of thigh from lateral to medial side.*

Action – *flexes hip and knee, e.g. when sitting cross-legged.*

Semitendinosus (hamstrings) – *down posterior medial side of thigh.*

Action – *extends thigh, flexes leg at knee.*

Quadriceps extensor – *on the front of the thigh.*

Action – *opposite movement to hamstrings.*

External oblique – *extends laterally down the side of the abdomen.*

Action – *compresses abdomen, twists trunk.*

Internal oblique – *extends laterally down the side of the front of the abdomen.*

Action – *compresses abdomen, twists trunk, works with the external oblique.*

Rectus abdominis – *runs down the entire length of the front of the abdomen (divided into four sections).*

Action – *an important muscle for maintaining posture, draws front of pelvis upwards.*

Transverse abdominis – *laterally on front of abdomen.*

    Action – compresses abdomen.

Erector spinae – *found medially on the posterior surface of neck, thorax and abdomen.*

    Action – extends the spine, holds body upright.

Latissimus dorsi – *runs down back of lower thorax and lumbar region.*

    Action – draws shoulders downwards and backwards, adducts and rotates arm, helps pull body up.

The Body

4

Preparations

WHAT YOU SHOULD KNOW BEFORE YOU START TO EXERCISE

The Pilates-based Body Maintenance exercises require total concentration and focus. This makes it particularly important to find a time and place to do them where you know you will not be disturbed. This might mean switching off the telephone and ridding yourself of other distractions so that you're not interrupted. You will also need to create a specific space for yourself where you can exercise. Most of us do not have the facilities to have our own private gyms! You may, however, find an area in your house that becomes your own retreat. It helps if you get into the right frame of mind. Do this by thinking – this is *my* time, I am creating a space within my house, within my environment, to work on *my* body for *myself*, without distractions.

When to Exercise

The exercises in the core exercise programme can be done at any time of the day. You might find that you prefer to do them in the early evening, to help you unwind and loosen tight muscles after a busy day. If you find it difficult to get going in the mornings, a 15-minute session first thing may be just what you need.

Clothes

Ideally, you should wear clothing in which you can exercise comfortably, such as leggings, shorts and a T-shirt, or leotard top. Don't wear anything which will restrict your movements. Opt for natural fibres like cotton, which are cooler. You can exercise wearing socks or in bare feet. If you are concerned about slipping, put on a pair of trainers. Take off any jewellery which might get in the way.

Equipment

Having picked a suitable spot in which to exercise, try to create adequate
room. This may mean moving the furniture and clearing away any clutter.
Before you start, check the floor for any sharp objects or stray pins. Most of
the exercises require little or no equipment. It is essential however to work
on a padded surface or a mat. This will protect your spine and prevent any
bruising against a hard floor. It is probably worth investing in a proper sports
mat. Alternatively, you can work on a folded, synthetic blanket. This should
be about five or six feet long and a foot wide. Some of the exercises involve
using props such as a chair, sofa or dresser. Always make sure these are
secure. If an exercise indicates that you need a couple of light handweights
and you don't have any, you can substitute cans of beans. If possible, try
exercising in front of a full-length mirror. This will enable you to check
what you are doing.

WHICH EXERCISES?

With the Pilates Body Maintenance Exercise Programme it is really
important to *always* start your exercise routine with the pelvic tilts and the
abdominal exercises, because you will be working from a strong centre.
Even when working your arms and legs everything is controlled from the
centre. Thus, if you are standing and doing a calf stretch, you should be
thinking about the location of your stomach, spine and shoulders. As well as
doing some basic abdominal work, each session you do should also
incorporate stretches after the relevant strengthening exercises. You can
then do upper and lower body work on alternate days.

If you have a specific medical condition such as repetitive strain injury (carpal
tunnel syndrome), scoliosis, sciatica or a bad back, only do those exercises
that are recommended for that particular condition (see pages 163–8).

Sequence of Exercises

1) *Do all the pelvic tilt and abdominal exercises at the beginning.*
2) *Proceed to do the back exercises.*
3) *Leg exercises and stretches.*
4) *All upper body exercises and stretches.*

Read all the instructions carefully. Remember the breathing instructions.

Continue to add exercises each day as you feel more comfortable. Use your own judgement. If you are unsure do the pelvic tilts and abdominal exercises, then add to them. If you feel any discomfort in your back during any particular exercise, you still have insufficient core strength to do it.

In Pilates-based Body Maintenance there are a number of basic safety rules:

- *Always do stretches after the relevant strengthening exercises.*
- *Do not attempt to do too much too soon. Increase the number of repetitions gradually.*
- *If you feel nauseous, fatigued or extremely breathless – stop.*
- *If you have any chest pains* (especially *when accompanied by pain in the arm, neck, shoulders and jaw) – stop exercising* immediately *and seek medical help.*
- *If exercise leaves you unnaturally tired, check with your doctor.*
- *The neck is a sensitive area of the body. If you cannot remember if you have worked this area or not, it is better not to do any further repetitions.*
- *Always make sure that there is something you can hold on to for support when doing the balancing exercises.*
- *If you experience back pain – stop.*
- *If your muscles start shaking – stop.*
- *Drink plenty of fluids afterwards, especially when it is hot.*

Before you embark on any new programme, it's a good idea to consult your doctor. A pre-exercise check-up is strongly advised if you are over 40 or have not been exercising regularly. *Always* seek the advice of a specialist if you have a known medical condition, are pregnant or have any chronic joint problems.

The
Exercise
Programme

The core exercises in this section will help you to tone and strengthen specific muscles in your arms, back, stomach, chest and legs. In time, as your body adapts, you will also start to look taller, slimmer and more youthful. In addition to improving your physical shape, strength and flexibility, some of these exercises will be very helpful if you suffer from any of the following medical conditions – scoliosis, repetitive strain injury (carpal tunnel syndrome), back pain and sciatica.

Before you attempt any of the exercises in the rest of the core programme, start with the following essential posture and balance exercises. It is best to do these in bare feet. If you've got a mirror – even better. That way, if you stand side-ways, you'll be able to keep an eye on what you're doing and make sure that it's correct.

PERFECT POSTURE – HOW TO LOOK INSTANTLY TALLER AND SLIMMER

Not sure if you're standing correctly? Then practice this position for a few minutes daily. After a while it will feel so natural that you no longer have to think about it.

Stand with your feet hip-width apart. Imagine that you're standing on sand. Your feet are relaxed. Think of your weight being over the middle of each foot, with your toes gently lengthening into the sand. Close your eyes and make a mental note of the following:

- *Don't sink back into your heels or lean forward. Keep your weight evenly distributed over your feet.*
- *Let your arms fall naturally in front of your body.*
- *Let your hands hang from the shoulders, totally loose and relaxed.*
- *Don't lock your knees. They should feel relaxed and not rigid.*

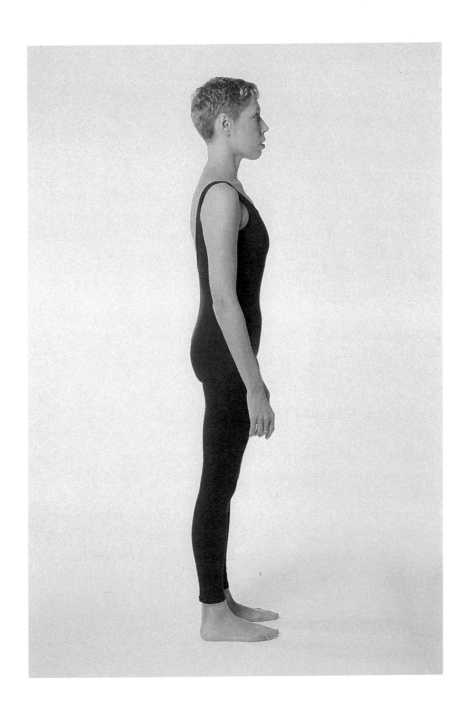

The Exercise Programme

- *Keep your inside thighs and bottom relaxed.*
- *Imagine that your head is like one of those nodding dogs in the back of car. It's not going backwards and forwards but resting directly upon your shoulders and rocking gently until it settles into a comfortable, neutral position.*
- *Think of the bones directly behind your ears. Try to imagine them 'reaching' towards the ceiling.*
- *Pull your stomach in, without tipping the pelvis forward. Think of a piece of string from your pubic bone to your navel. It is shortening as you pull up and in. Feel your tailbone drop – as if it is weighted to the floor. This will seem much easier after you've done more of the stretches to release the pelvic girdle.*
- *Keep the front of your thighs relaxed.*

Now your whole body is perfectly aligned – you should feel as if you are floating an inch off the ground.

38

EXERCISES FOR BETTER BALANCE

If you're worried about slipping, tripping or not being able to catch objects thrown towards you, your sense of balance is most probably poor. What seems to occur, as you get older or as a result of any injury, is that you lose your awareness of balance and your reflexes are no longer as sharp. This can cause great feelings of insecurity. Perhaps you begin to worry more about safety. We all know that the simplest of falls might have serious consequences. This is reflected in the body, which becomes stiff and constricted as a result. The easiest way to change this is to practise the following exercises every day. In time, you will start to feel lighter and more confident in the way you move.

For each of these exercises all the same rules as the 'perfect posture' exercise apply (see the checklist above).

Standing on One Leg

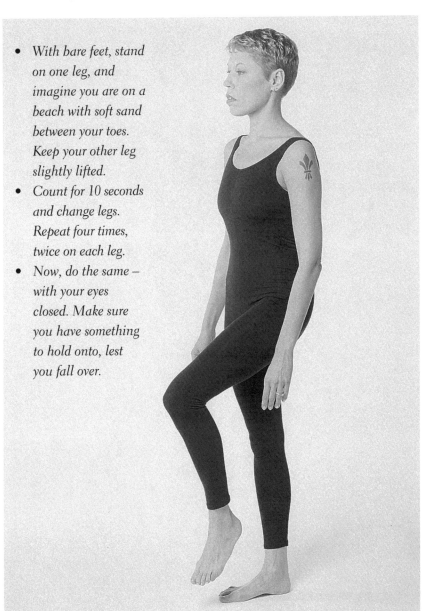

- *With bare feet, stand on one leg, and imagine you are on a beach with soft sand between your toes. Keep your other leg slightly lifted.*
- *Count for 10 seconds and change legs. Repeat four times, twice on each leg.*
- *Now, do the same – with your eyes closed. Make sure you have something to hold onto, lest you fall over.*

The Exercise Programme

Standing on One Leg on a Towel

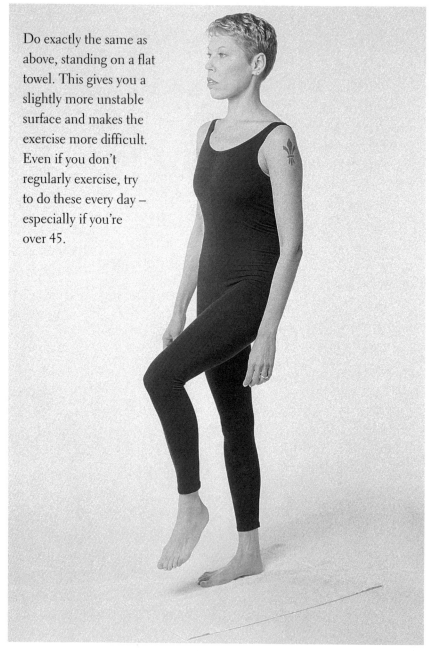

Do exactly the same as above, standing on a flat towel. This gives you a slightly more unstable surface and makes the exercise more difficult. Even if you don't regularly exercise, try to do these every day – especially if you're over 45.

Walking Backwards

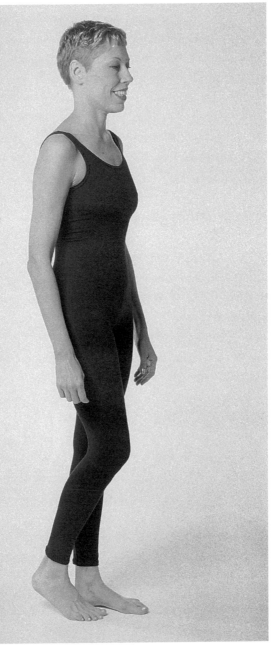

Start in the 'perfect posture' position and, with feet approximately an inch apart, start to walk backwards. Slowly drag your foot back, so that it never entirely leaves the floor. The easiest way to master this is to imagine that you are trying to remove some chewing gum from under your feet.

Look in the mirror – but do not look down at your feet.

This exercise is even more effective if you imagine you are walking on sand.

41

The Exercise Programme

BREATHING

Correct breathing is a very important facet of Pilates. By remembering to breathe properly, you'll find it becomes much easier to exercise. The problem is that most people don't breathe deeply enough. Breathing slowly and deeply is very energizing. It ensures there is sufficient oxygen circulating throughout the body.

It may sound obvious, but when you exercise do not hold your breath. It's better to breathe incorrectly than not at all. Practise the following exercise before you start any of the stomach work.

Basic Breathing Exercise

- *Lie on your back in a relaxed position, resting your head on a folded towel, with your knees bent.*
- *Place one hand on your stomach and, very gently, breathe in through your nose. Feel your lungs filling with oxygen and slowly expand and relax your stomach. Breathe out.*
- *With one finger on your pubic bone and one on your navel, try and shorten that gap as you breathe out, and flatten your stomach to your spine without tilting your pelvis.*
- *Breathe in again and feel that gap slightly expand.*
- *Breathe out. Imagine there is a piece of string or an elastic band that links your pubic bone to your navel. Very gently feel it pulling up and in. This will get all three sets of stomach muscles working, including your oblique muscles, which will tighten your waist.*

Make sure you breathe slowly and deeply. One of the main rules of Pilates is to breathe out on the point of effort. If in doubt, particularly on the stretches – breathe naturally.

When you breathe in your stomach gently expands. However, it shouldn't swell in an exaggerated way. Try and think of your ribcage expanding gently to the sides so that you're not just breathing into your throat and upper chest.

When you begin this exercise programme and you start to breathe properly you might feel a bit dizzy. As you are learning to breathe more deeply, you are taking in more oxygen – which can make you feel light-headed.

BASIC ABDOMINAL AND BACK EXERCISES

These basic abdominal and back exercises are good for conditioning, toning and strengthening. They're also good for anyone with a bad back, sciatica or scoliosis. If you have any of these problems you need to do abdominal and back work, but do not attempt any of the advanced exercises at first.

It's better to do these exercises either lying on a towel or on an exercise mat. As you're lying on your back, you may want to place a folded towel under your head. This will help lengthen your neck. If you're not sure about this, try it with and without a small folded towel and see which is more comfortable.

Repeat *each* exercise 10 times. Do the stretches in sets of four.

1. Pelvic Tilt

The Pelvic Tilt is a preparation exercise that warms up the back. It's a good starting point, whatever part of the programme you plan to do.

Lie on your back, with your knees bent and parallel, about 6–8 inches apart. Arms should be resting at your sides, with palms facing the floor. This helps to lengthen your neck. Breathe in, then breathe out and gently relax your back into the floor. When you do this, do not press your back too strongly to the ground so that you lose your natural curve. Do not allow your back to arch to the point that it lifts off the floor. This is called the *neutral spine position* and it is slightly different for everybody (see p.19). There is no point in trying to force your back down. Try very hard not to tense your buttock muscles during this exercise.

As you breathe out gently tilt your pelvis forward and roll your lower back off the floor – one vertebra at a time, as you 'peel' your back off the mat (see p.21). Breathe in, keeping your neck long, and very slowly roll all the way down breathing out. Keep your feet relaxed on the floor and imagine that your toes are 'lengthening' away.

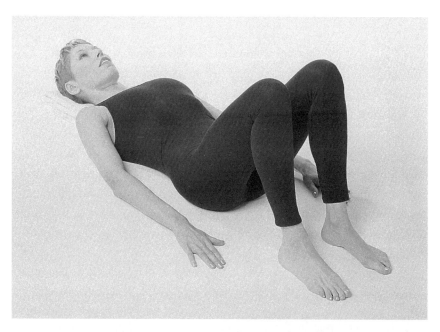

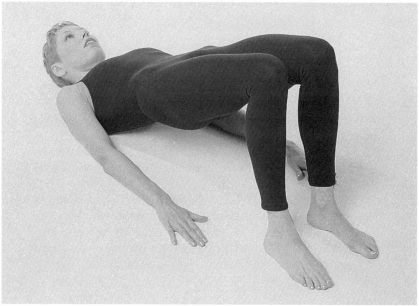

The Exercise Programme

2. Preparation for abdominals

This is a preparation for the abdominal exercises. It will wake up your stomach muscles and prepare you for the more difficult exercises.

Lie as before – with a relaxed back and long neck, without tucking the pelvis under. Take either a small cushion or folded towel and place it between your thighs. Very gently breathe in through your nose. As you breathe out, feel your stomach muscles pulling down to the floor. Think of them pulling up and into your spine. Hold your breath and count to four. Squeeze the towel or cushion with your thighs. You can put your fingers on your stomach if you wish so that you can feel the muscles you are working.

As you breathe in through your nose, feel your stomach gently expand into your fingers. As you breathe out, feel your stomach pull away from your fingers. Feel your lower abdominal muscles working. Think of working on the transverse and the rectus abdominis muscles first, and the obliques second (see the figure on p.24). Repeat 10 times.

Watchpoints

- Don't let your pelvis lift off the floor. This will 'shorten' the neck. Watch that your stomach doesn't 'bloat'. Instead, make sure that on the point of relaxation – when you breathe in – the stomach gently lifts. As you breathe out you should feel your stomach pull up and in, away from the pubic bone.

- Most people naturally want to breathe in and pull their stomach muscles in – this is a mistake. As you breathe in, you gently soften the muscles as they flow out into your fingers. As you breathe out the stomach pulls away from the fingers. Think of it as pulling 'up and in'. This will help you focus on your lower abdominals – strengthening and toning that area.

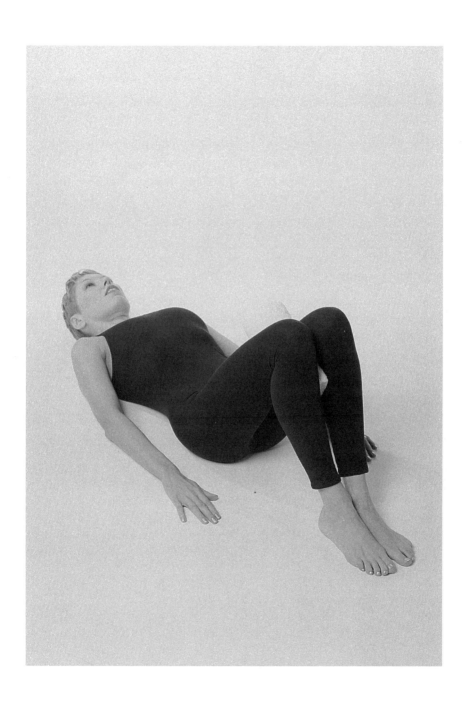

The Exercise Programme

3. Working the Lower Abdominal Muscles

Lie in the same position as above, knees bent. Place your hands on your hipbones. This helps to stabilize your pelvis. Begin with the right leg. Keep your left leg completely still. Very gently breathe in and let your right knee open sideways. As you breathe out feel the resistance. Bring the leg back to the other one – breathing out and pulling your stomach in. Change legs. Now, breathing in, open the left leg to the side. Exhale and slowly close. Repeat 10 times, alternating legs each time.

Watchpoints

- Think of the muscles between your navel and your pubic bone as a fan. As you inhale and the knee opens to the side – the fan opens. As you exhale, the muscles tighten and the fan closes.

- Don't tilt the pelvis, and make sure that the supporting side is stable.

- Don't press your back into the mat.

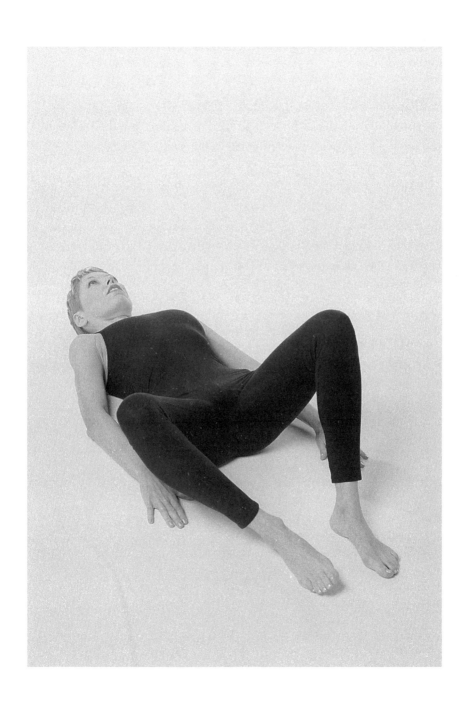

The Exercise Programme

4. Working the Lower Abdominal Muscles

This slightly harder version of exercise 3 is very straightforward. Interlace your hands behind your head. (This will help prevent you from straining the muscles in your neck.) Slide them high up behind your skull. Do not let them slip to the neck. Keep thumbs on either side of your spine.

Lift your elbows so that you can just see them out of the corner of your eye – *without* moving your head. When you can see your elbows peripherally you know that your arms are in the right place. Very gently exhale and 'float' your head and shoulders off the mat. Hold that position and repeat exercise 3 above. Repeat the exercise 10 times, five times on each side.

> ### Watchpoint
>
> As you lift your head, your focus shouldn't change – so you don't shorten your neck. If you shorten your neck you may tip your pelvis. This makes it very hard to work your lower abdominal muscles. You may also place a strain on your lower back and your body will be incorrectly aligned.

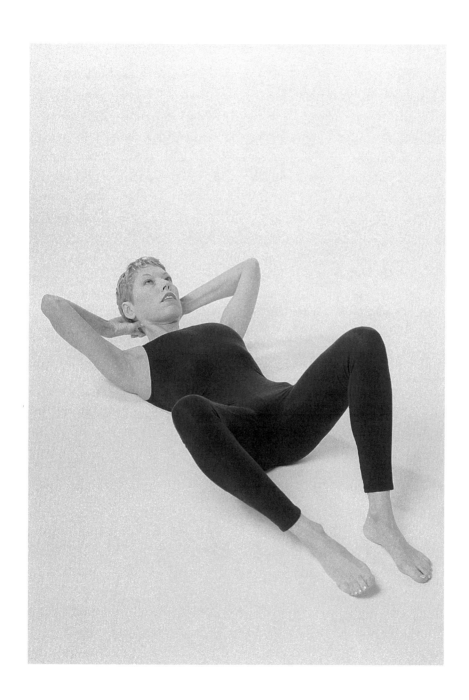

The Exercise Programme

5. Basic Abdominal Curl

This exercise uses exactly the same position as exercise 4, although the knee does not fan out. All the same rules apply. Lift your elbows up where you can see them in peripheral vision. Keep looking at the ceiling and gently breathe in through your nose. Relax the abdomen – but do not 'bloat' it out. As you breathe out, gently lift your head and shoulders off the mat. Only go as high as you can. Do not strain your neck to hold that position. Breathe in as you go back down again.

Watchpoint

As you breathe out, imagine that a piece of string is pulling you up from your pubic bone and under your rib cage. Pause until all three sets of abdominal muscles go 'up and in' – and flatten.

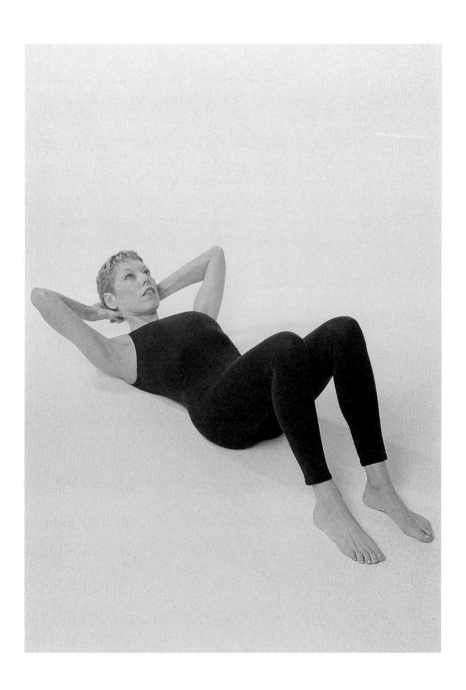

53

The Exercise Programme

6. Single Leg Stretch

This stomach exercise is a simple single leg stretch. It is the first really co-ordinated exercise. It is a simple and basic exercise – which is not the same as saying it is easy.

Start in the same position as exercise 3 and interlace your hands behind your head. Lift your head and shoulders gently off the mat. As you breathe out, slide your right leg down, an inch off the floor. Breathe in, putting your head down and bringing your right leg back up. Breathe out, and slide your left leg down, an inch off the floor. Repeat 10 times, alternating the legs.

Watchpoints

- Many people make the mistake of exhaling before curling forward. If you do this, you will not get the same benefit. You exhale as you do the exercise.

- Remember to keep looking at that same point on the ceiling. If you pull your chin into your chest you may strain your neck and won't get the results you want.

The following two exercises are demonstrated with a partner. Therefore if you wish to work with a partner one of you can hold the legs. Alternatively, if you're working alone, you can put your legs against a wall.

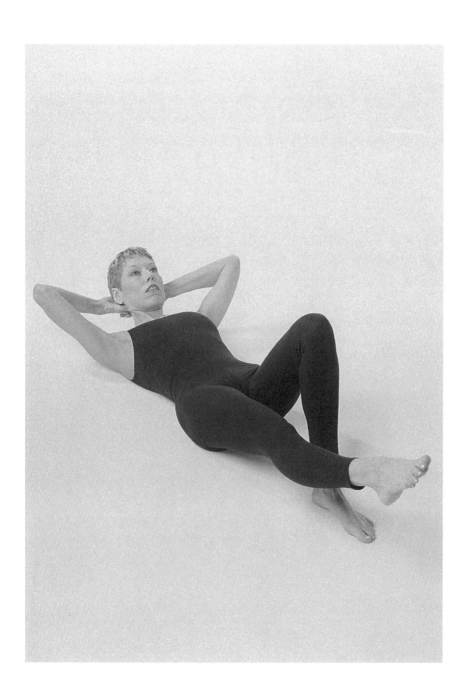

The Exercise Programme

7. Exercise with Partner

Lying down, put your legs up against the wall, so that your tailbone is completely relaxed to the floor. If your bottom is slightly lifted off the floor – you're too close. On the other hand, if you're too far away, you will not feel supported. Make sure your legs are comfortably rotated outwards – so that they're gently turned out in the sockets. Keep knees slightly bent. Now do exactly the same as in exercise 5 – a very simple sit up. It is more difficult because your legs are on the wall.

With your hands behind your head, legs comfortably supported by the wall and tailbone heavy, lift your elbows and imagine a star on the ceiling. Breathe out and lift your head and shoulders. As you breathe in, relax down. Exhale as you lift. This exercise will work the slightly higher abdominal muscles. Repeat 10 times.

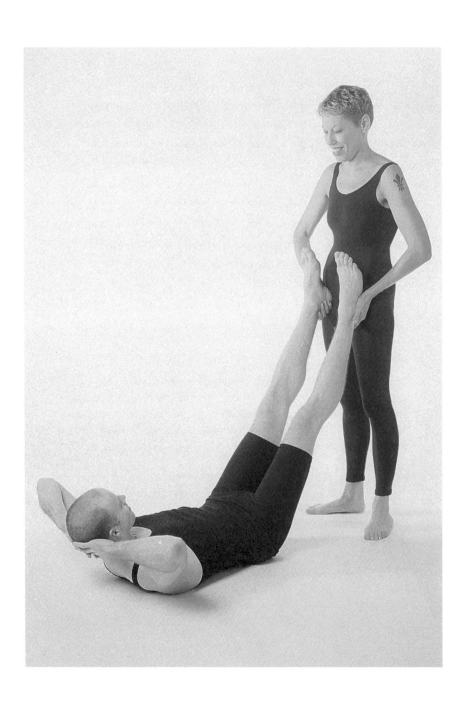

The Exercise Programme

8. Exercise with Partner

This exercise is very similar but it has got a 'twist'. Most twisting exercises actually work the waist – the obliques. The internal and external obliques are essential for core stability and the mobility of the spine. If you want to have a strong stomach and strong back you must have core stability. If your muscles are too tight, you will have problems twisting and mobilizing your spine.

Remain in exactly the same position as before in exercise 7, breathe out and take a very small twist, easing the right elbow to the left knee. Don't get so high that you feel any strain in the neck. Breathe in as you release down. Exhale as you twist to the other side.

Watchpoints

- If you're unsure about this exercise, you can place one hand on the side you're working. As you breathe out, feel those waist muscles pulling away from your fingers. If they're pushing into your fingers, you've lifted too high. This may happen because your stomach muscles aren't strong enough or your back is too tight.

- With any of the abdominal exercises, it's important to lift only the head and shoulders as high as the point when your stomach flattens to your spine. If you lift too high and your stomach doesn't go in – you are building muscle. You might want to do this but you won't want to build muscle which will protrude. Perfect abdominal muscles are strong, firm and flat to the spine. They act as support for the spine and the internal organs. They're also meant to look taut and glamorous.

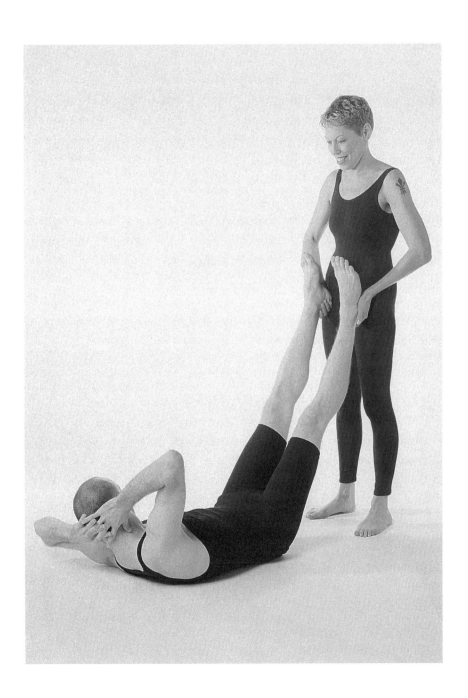

The Exercise Programme

9. Advanced Single Leg Stretch

This is the most difficult exercise in the programme, because it is an exercise with both legs off the ground. If you have any back injuries at all – don't do it until you feel strong enough.

Bend both knees into the chest and allow your tailbone to be relaxed and heavy. Your hands are linked behind your head as before. Look at your star in the ceiling and breathe out. Let your head and shoulders 'float' off the ground – depending on how much mobility you have.

Inhale. Exhale and stretch one leg out, pulling your stomach into the spine. Inhale and bring the leg back. Exhale and extend the other leg. Do five stretches on each leg. If you wish you may relax at the end and do another set. Only take the leg as low as the point when your back does not arch away from the floor. The lower the leg, the harder the exercise.

SIDE STRETCHES AND SIDE LIFTS

The next three exercises are also abdominal exercises but they are done lying on your side. These are called side stretches and side lifts. They are particularly good for the waist obliques. The same rules apply as to all the abdominal exercises. It doesn't matter which side you lie on to start with. Do all the exercises in sets of 10.

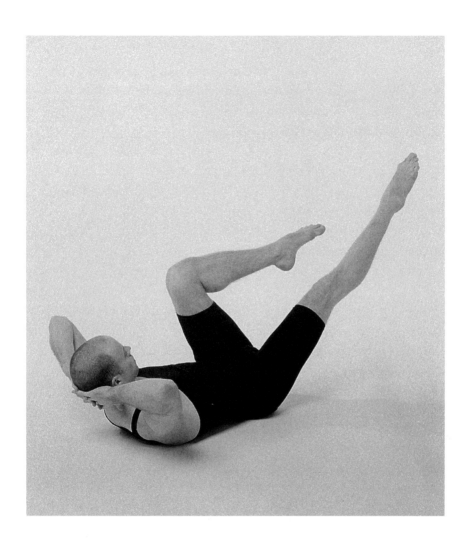

The Exercise Programme

10. Side Stretch

Lie on your side, arm stretched out in line with your body, resting on the floor, palm down. Place your other hand on the floor in front of you, for balance. If your neck doesn't feel comfortable, place a folded towel between your ear and your shoulder.

Think of your ear 'lengthening' along the arm, so that you're looking directly ahead of you. The hips are stacked one directly over the other so that your pelvis is level, not tilted. It's very common to let the top hip rock forward. Glance down your body without moving your head. If you can't see your feet, they are too far behind you. If you feel any strain in your back, the first thing you should do is move your feet further forward.

Breathe in to prepare. Breathe out and lift your legs about four inches off the ground. Keep your feet gently flexed. You want to straighten the back of your legs. Feel the energy pushing through your heels as you lift. Breathe in as you lower. Do 10 each side.

Watchpoints

- If you are unsure about this position, do it with your back against the wall. You can then feel how far your legs have to come forward to feel your middle back against the wall.

- Stretch your legs as far as you can without locking your knees. The knees are lengthened away, but slightly relaxed. If you're not sure about locking your knees or stretching your knees it's always better to have them slightly released.

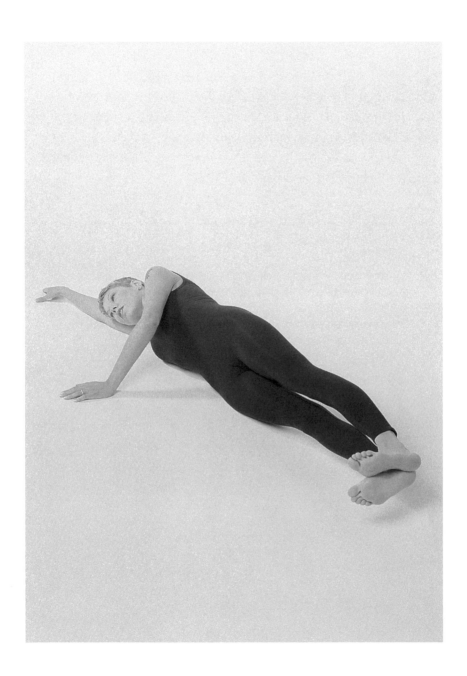

The Exercise Programme

11. Side Stretch

The next exercise is simply a harder version of the one before – so all the same rules apply. Use a towel if you need to. Relax your top arm and shoulder. With flexed feet breathe out and think of your legs floating off the ground. Hold this position and breathe in. Breathe out and lift the top leg. Bring the leg back, breathe in, and slowly lower both legs to the ground and relax. Do 10 repetitions on each side.

Watchpoints

- It's really important for this exercise that you never allow one leg to become longer than the other. You don't want an imbalance in your pelvis.

- Correct breathing is vital. If you feel any strain in your back, try doing the exercise with your legs further forward.

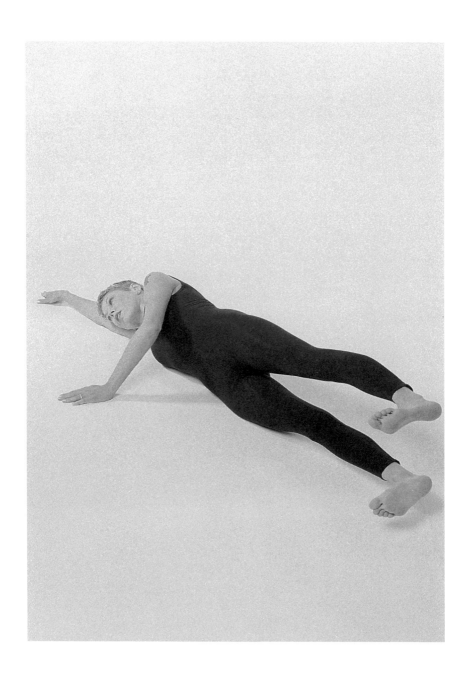

The Exercise Programme

12. Side Lift

The next exercise is more difficult and you need to be reasonably fit to try it. Don't attempt it if you have any back injuries.

Lie on your side, with your elbow directly under your shoulder, your palm flat on the floor. Keep your legs in a straight line with your ankles crossed. It helps if can place your feet against a hard surface – e.g., a skirting board, or bottom of a sofa. This will give you a bit of resistance and help you get off the ground. All the same rules on alignment apply as in exercise 10. Keep your shoulder and elbow in line. As you breathe out, lift, pushing down through the supporting arm. The other arm lifts up to a right angle in line with the shoulder. Come back down again and relax. With this exercise begin by doing it four times on each side and slowly build up to 10. This will give you a strong, toned and, hopefully, very trim waist.

66

BACK EXERCISES

We now begin the back sequence. Back exercises are vital for a strong stomach and back because both sets of muscles support the torso. Without a strong back you don't have a strong body.

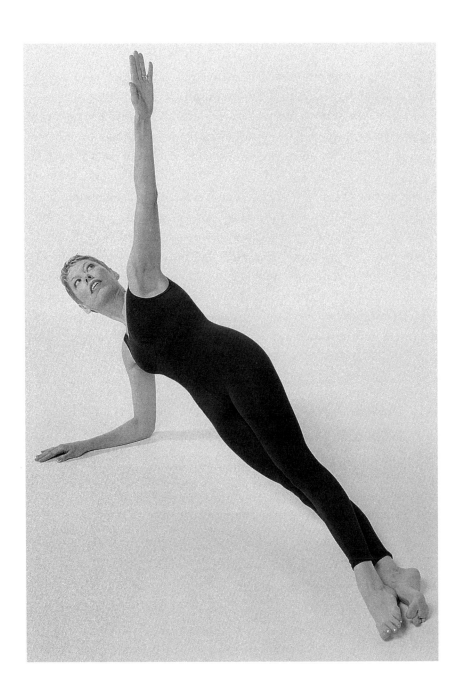

The Exercise Programme

13. Cat Stretch

A cat stretch is done on your hands and knees. Make a square of your body. Keep your hands under your shoulders, fingers facing forwards and with your hands a shoulder-width apart. Knees should be hip-width apart. If your knees feel a bit uncomfortable, just fold up a towel and put it under them. Place your feet gently on the floor and don't lock your elbows at any point.

As you breathe out, drop your chin to your chest and curl your stomach into the spine. Press your upper back to the ceiling, trying not to rock back and forth. As you breathe in, your tailbone lifts towards the ceiling, your chest presses to the floor and your head gently lifts. Breathe out and reverse the position. After 10 repetitions, relax your bottom onto your heels and just breathe. This is called the 'relaxation position' (see end of sequence, p.80). You can do this relaxation at the end of the sequence of back exercises, or at the end of each back exercise.

Watchpoints

- Don't lock your elbows.

- Don't lift your head too high or you may strain your neck.

- As you press your chest down to the floor (in the reverse exercise), if you feel any pinching in your lower back you'll know you've gone too far.

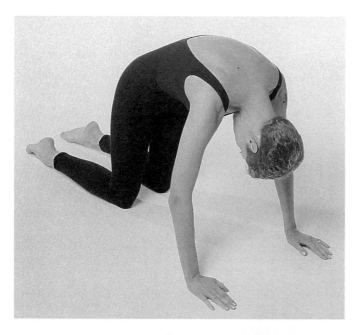

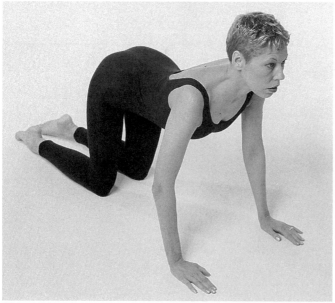

The Exercise Programme

14. Back Strengthening

Lie on your stomach with your feet relaxed. Your arms should be facing forwards and be just wider than your shoulders, which are relaxed. Keep your neck 'long' by looking down. Keep looking down as you gently press your hips and elbows into the floor and pull your stomach in. Gently, lift your head up (keep it independent of the body), focusing your eyes on the same point. Make sure you keep your feet on the floor. Breathe in, and gently come down. Feel your buttocks contract slightly. Do not contract them too much – otherwise you're using your buttock muscles and not the stomach. Engaging the abdominals helps to strengthen your back and lift your body.

As you breathe out and lift, imagine that the crown of your head is going forward towards the wall in front of you. Do not lift your head towards the ceiling. Ideally, you want as little pressure on the hands as possible. Relax your fingers and feel your shoulder blades releasing. Relax down again.

Watchpoints

- As you breathe out and lift, you should be able to get your fingers between your stomach and the floor.

- Whenever you do a back exercise, each time you breathe out, your stomach goes into the spine (just as in the earlier abdominal exercises). If you lift too high and you feel your back shortening, you've gone too far.

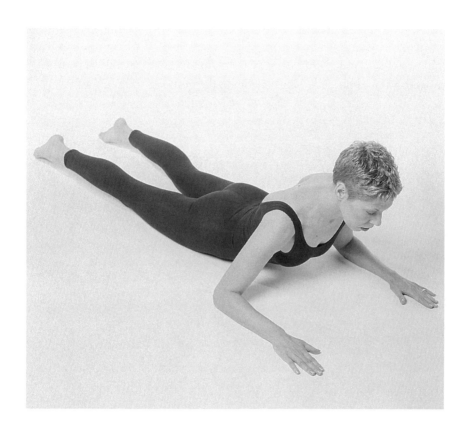

The Exercise Programme

15. Back Strengthening

This exercise is exactly the same as above, except that this time, as you breathe out and lift, your hands 'float' off the ground.

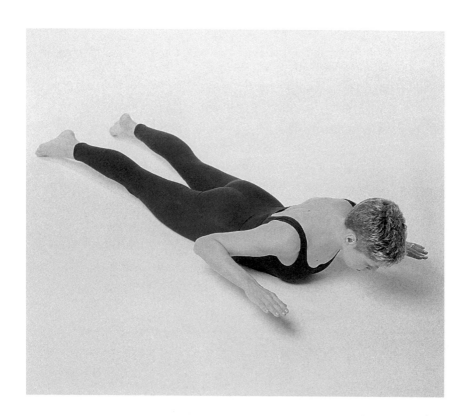

The Exercise Programme

16. Alternate Arm and Leg Stretch for the Back

This works your stomach and your back.

Lying on your stomach imagine yourself in the shape of a rather small starfish. Your arms are slightly wider than your shoulders. Look down at the floor. Make sure your legs are comfortably apart and rotated slightly outwards. Don't force it though, simply lie there and just let your legs relax into their natural position. Exhale and let your left leg and right arm gently float off the ground. Feel your stomach doing all the work. Breathe in and lower. Exhale as you change sides. Make sure that as your stomach goes in your tailbone drops. As you breathe, don't grip your bottom. Again, keep your legs straight and shoulders relaxed. Your arms and legs should be at the same height. Repeat 10 times, alternating between sides.

74

Watchpoint

Don't shorten your neck, grip your bottom, or lift your arm and leg too high. Don't think of 'lifting' – you should be 'lengthening' your arm and leg. The idea here is to do a diagonal stretch that strengthens and mobilizes the big back muscle between the base of one shoulder blade and the top of the opposite buttock.

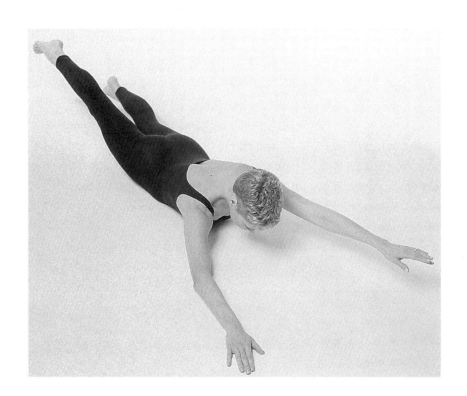

The Exercise Programme

17. Kneeling Arm and Leg Stretch

This exercise helps improve balance.

Assume the same position as the cat stretch (exercise 13). The spine is neutral and stomach gently in. Imagine someone's hand on your stomach. Breathe out, and let your right arm and left leg gently float away. Don't lift too high. To avoid this, position something like a kitchen roll across the base of your spine. If you lift too high, it will fall off. Keep your pelvis neutral, so that you don't tilt from side to side. Keep looking at the same point on the floor, so that you don't shorten your neck. Relax back into the starting position. Repeat, alternating arms and legs for 10 repetitions.

Watchpoint

If this exercise feels too difficult at the onset, you can start by lifting one arm, or one leg only.

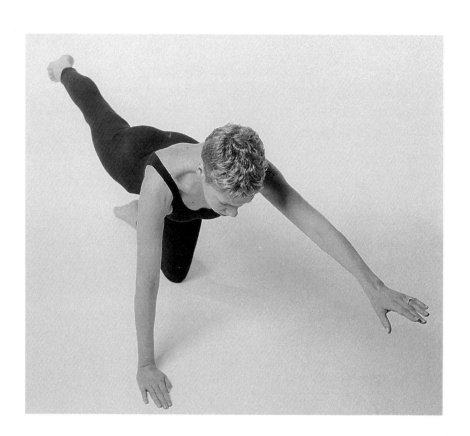

The Exercise Programme

18. The Swan – Advanced Back Exercise

All the same rules apply as in exercise 16 (alternate arm and leg stretch).
Once again imagine you are a small starfish, lying on your front, with your
arms and legs comfortably apart. As you breathe out, simultaneously lift
both arms and both legs to the same height. Keep looking down
throughout, and pull your stomach into your spine until you feel your
tailbone drop.

Watchpoints

- Make sure that as your stomach goes in, your pelvis relaxes back; as you
  breathe, don't grip your bottom.

- Again, keep your legs straight. If you bend your knees the exercise won't be
  effective.

- Keep shoulders relaxed, stomach in, legs and arms straight. Your arms and
  legs should be at the same height.

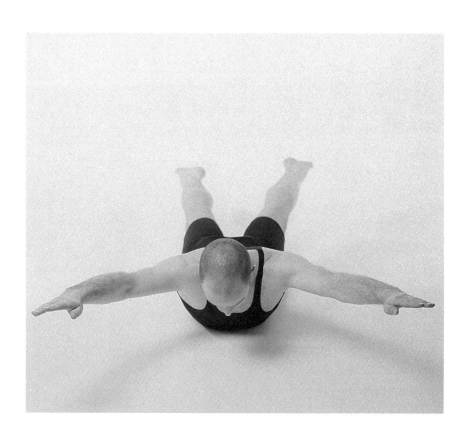

The Exercise Programme

19. Relaxation Position – Child's Pose

Do this at the end of the back exercise sequence.

Sit back down on your heels with your arms close to your sides. Gently pull your head into your chest and curl yourself into a small 'ball' until your forehead touches the ground. Hold for a few seconds.

LEGS

The following exercises will help to strengthen, tone and condition your legs. They will help to make your legs more shapely – many people tend to have over-developed quads, weak inside thighs and tight, but not strong, hamstrings.

Any of the following exercises can be done with ankle weights. However, don't use anything heavier than one kilo. You want to tone and lengthen muscles, not build them up.

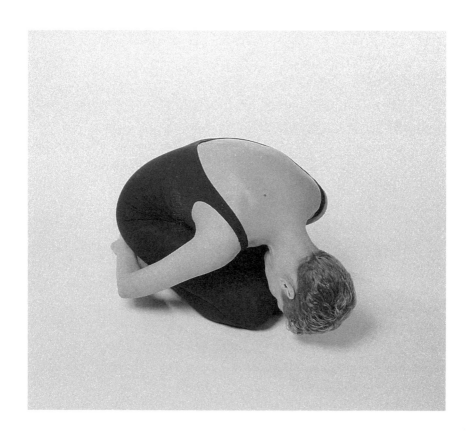

The Exercise Programme

20. Inside Thigh Lift

This exercise will help tone flabby, inside thighs.

You can do this lying on your side, either with your hand supporting your head, or with your arm completely flat. If you choose to keep your arm flat, it may feel more comfortable to put a towel between your arm and ear. Your top leg should be forward, in front of the body. If this feels awkward, place a pillow under your knee. The other hand is in front of you. The underneath leg (the one that is working) needs to be slightly forward, with your foot gently flexed. Again, don't lock your knee, but pull up the muscles, so that your leg is straight. If your legs are not straight, you'll be working your ankle and your foot, much more than your inside thigh.

Breathe out, lift your leg and hold. Then slowly lower it. Don't lift your leg too high. Think of your leg going 'away', not up – as you want to lengthen and strengthen your muscles, not have them contracted and tight. As you lift and breathe out, your stomach pulls in, just like in the earlier stomach exercises. The energy is through the heel, working your inside thigh. Do 10 on each side.

> **Watchpoint**
>
> It's important to remember that, in all the leg exercises, the instigator is your stomach. This means you should feel your abdominal muscles working. The same applies to all the upper body exercises.

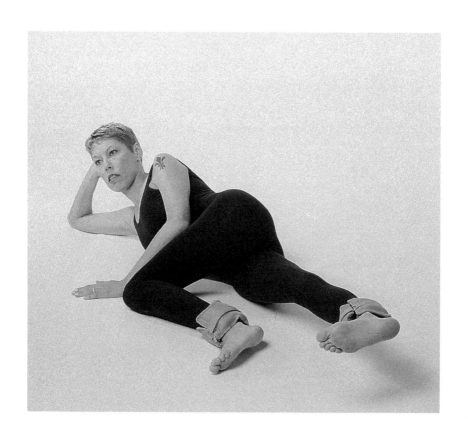

The Exercise Programme

21. Inside Thigh Circles

Assume the same position as in exercise 20. Gently point your foot. Breathe out and lift your leg. Slowly circle the leg in each direction. As you circle the leg, don't think of going up and down. Think of going out and away, so that you're almost touching the floor, as if you're circling around a fifty pence piece.

Do 10 little circles each way on each leg.

Watchpoint

The knee is gently pulled up, the leg is reaching away, and you're circling down and away – not up.

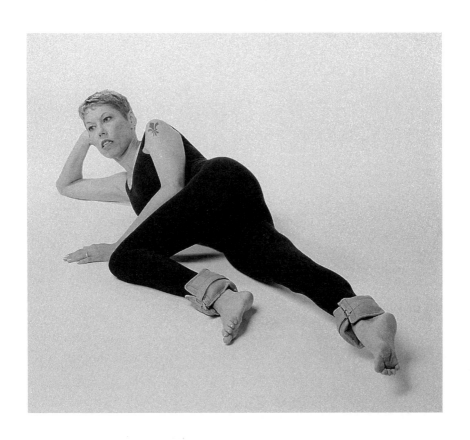

The Exercise Programme

22. Outer Thigh Lift

To work the outer thighs and buttocks.

Take up the same position as before, only this time your underneath leg is bent comfortably in front of you. The top leg is straight, flexed and very slightly forward. If you've got any doubts about your back arching, you can lean against a wall.

The top leg should start the exercise at hip height. Very gently breathe out and lift the leg about six inches. Don't turn your toes towards the ceiling. Keep your foot facing forward, gently flexed. When you breathe out and lift – focus on the outer thigh and the back of the leg.

Do 10 on each side.

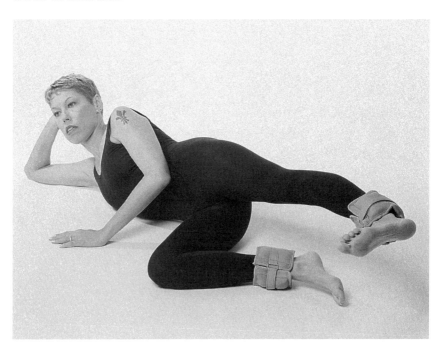

23. Outer Thighs and Buttocks

Start this exercise in the same position as exercise 22, but with both legs on the ground. Make sure your top heel is in line with your hip. Very gently breathe out and bring your leg forward, so that it's in line with the other knee. Breathe in, and lift. Breathe out, and lower and take leg back. This is quite a demanding exercise, so start with five on each side, then gradually build up to 10.

Watchpoints

- As you breathe out, and pull your leg forward, don't swing it. Think of your leg as a 'resistance', so that it is the stomach that is bringing your leg forward, up, down and back, as you tone the back of the thigh. Keep it in line with the other knee. Your hip stays back, your stomach stays in.

- If you find you get cramp in your hip, this exercise might not be for you.

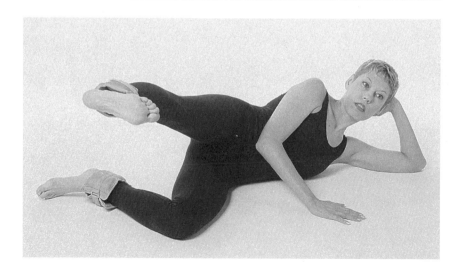

24. Outer Thighs and Buttocks

In the same position as before (exercise 23), bend both knees, so that they are comfortably in front of you. Gently flex your feet. Lift the top leg, as if you're opening a fan. Then very gently breathe out, and squeeze the top leg to straight. As you breathe in, make a small bend in the knee. Breathe out and squeeze to straight. Remember – the emphasis is not on the bend, but on the squeeze. If you do a big bend, you'll be working your calves, not your bottom. Do 10 on each side.

> **Watchpoint**
>
> If you get cramp, this indicates that your muscles are fatigued and it is best to stop.

The following exercises are all done lying on the stomach. They can all be done with one kilo ankle weights.

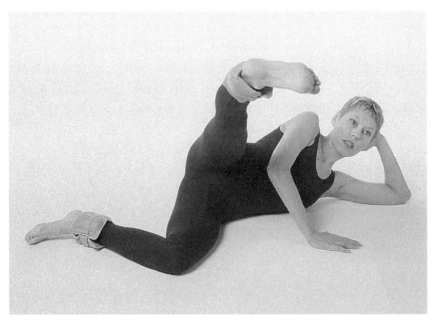

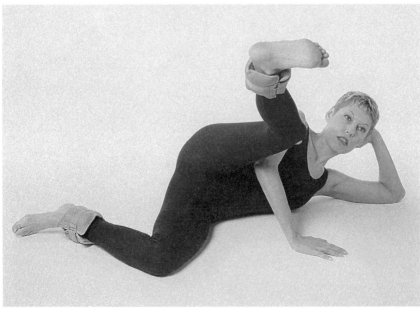

The Exercise Programme

25. Hamstring Toner and Strengthener

Lying on your stomach, your head should be comfortably relaxed on your hands. If you prefer, keep your arms at your sides. Do whichever feels more comfortable. Keep your shoulders relaxed. Very gently 'grip' your bottom. As you do so, you should feel your stomach going in and your tailbone drop. Inhaling, bend your right leg and flex your foot. Then and gently exhale and straighten, keeping the buttocks squeezed at all times. Repeat 10 times then change legs. (The bend on this exercise is not important – it's just a preparation.)

The next two exercises are similar, except for the position of the foot.

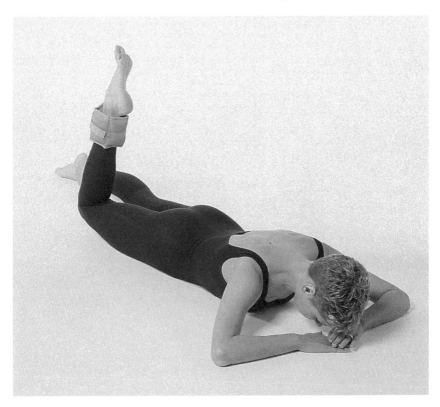

26. Bottom Toner

Assume the same position on your stomach as above. With a straight leg, hip down, stomach in, keeping foot relaxed, very gently breathe out and lift the leg up. Then slowly bring it down. This works the buttock muscles which are just under the cheek. Do 10 repetitions on each leg.

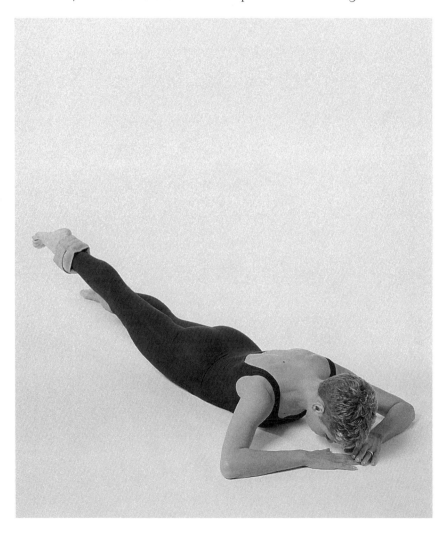

27. Bottom Toner

This is exactly the same as above, except this time as you breathe out and lift, keep your foot softly flexed. Repeat 10 times on one leg and then the other.

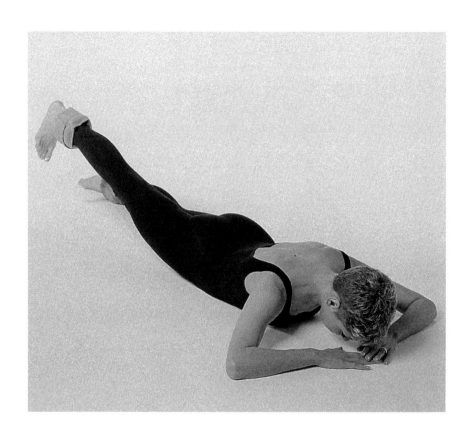

The Exercise Programme

28. Bottom Toner

This is the last exercise in this sequence – and all the same rules apply as above. Starting in the same position, this time you bend your leg and flex your foot as you lift. Keep your hip down, and foot, knee and ankle in line, as you breathe out and slowly squeeze towards the ceiling.

Repeat 10 times on one leg and then the other.

Watchpoints

- At no point in any of these three exercises should your hip-bones leave the mat.

- If you feel your back arch, place a rolled towel beneath your stomach.

LEG STRETCHES

It is vital that you do leg stretches after you've done any leg strengthening work. They are especially important if you have any back problems. If you've got a tight back, you may have tight legs. Sometimes it's difficult to know which comes first – a bad back and tight hamstrings, or tight hamstrings resulting in a bad back. Also, if you do have back problems you are likely to have a pelvic imbalance, which is often caused by over-tight gluteal muscles, hip flexors and quadriceps – so that your pelvis is not in line. If you can get your body in line, you'll feel much more comfortable, and you will avoid a lot of problems.

Hold all stretches for 30 seconds.

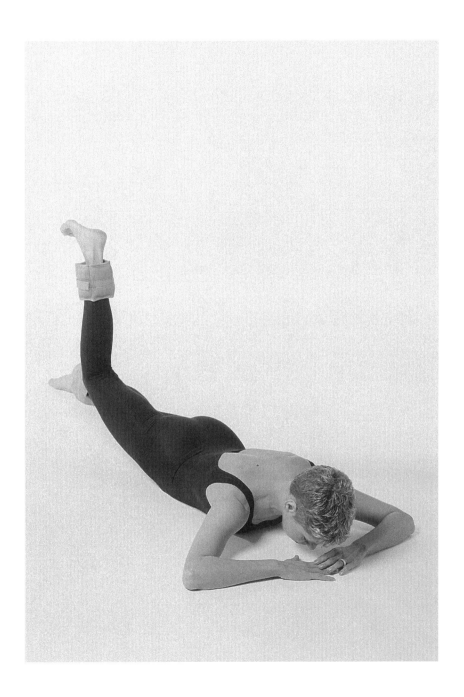

The Exercise Programme

29. Back and Hip – Gluteal Stretch

Lying down on your back, cross your knees, hold onto your ankles, and very gently pull your heels into your bottom. Do this for 30 seconds with the right leg on top, then 30 seconds with the left leg on top. Repeat four times in total.

Watchpoints

- Don't let your bottom lift – it should stay 'weighted' to the ground.

- Don't hold onto your feet – hold onto your ankles.

- If it feels more comfortable, place a towel under your head.

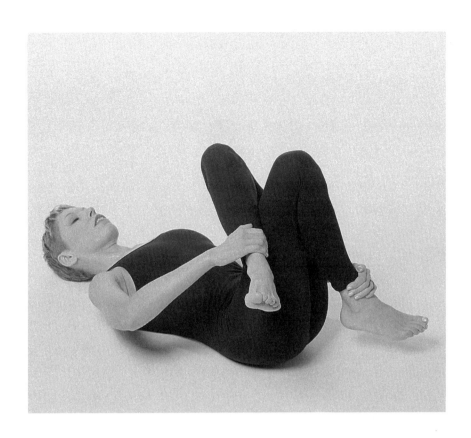

The Exercise Programme

30. Back and Hip – Gluteal Stretch

This is a slightly more advanced version of the above exercise. It will help to release the hips.

Lying on your back with your legs bent, very gently cross the right ankle over the left knee. Make sure it's the ankle, and not the toes. Gently, keeping your knee open, bend the leg into the chest and feel a stretch on the bent leg. Remember, on all the stretches, you should only feel a stretch on the working leg. Hold for 30 seconds, change legs and repeat four times.

Watchpoint

With both the above exercises, if you feel a strain in your back – stop. This means you're working your legs too hard.

The following exercises will stretch the quadricep muscles at front of your thighs. Hold all stretches for 30 seconds.

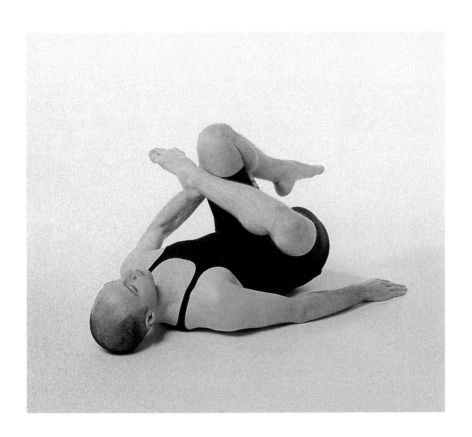

The Exercise Programme

31. Quadricep Stretch

Stand upright. Hold onto something if you feel you're losing your balance. Grasp one ankle and gently stretch the front of your thigh. Keep your knees in line (check in a mirror if you're not certain). Ensure that your stomach is in, and your tailbone dropped. You should be stretching from the hip flexor all the way down to the front of your thigh. Do not arch your back. Repeat four times, alternating legs.

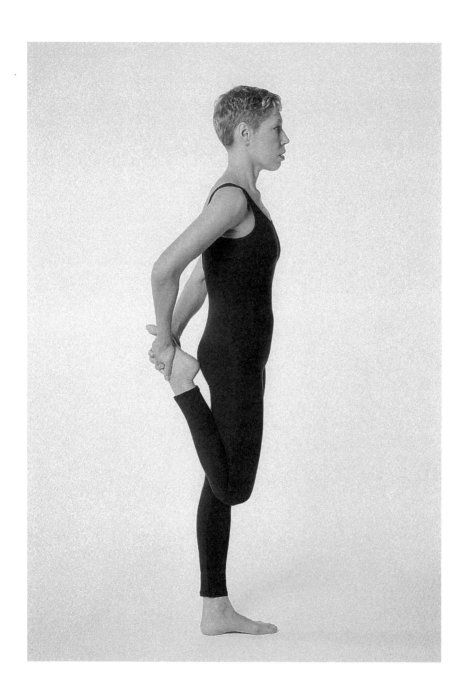

The Exercise Programme

32. Quadricep Stretch (advanced)

Kneel down on your right leg. Extend the left leg so that the knee is directly over the ankle. Gently pull your stomach in. Lean back slightly – without arching your back. Hold for 30 seconds. Repeat four times, alternating legs.

Watchpoint

If this stretch causes pain in your knee or your back – stop.

102

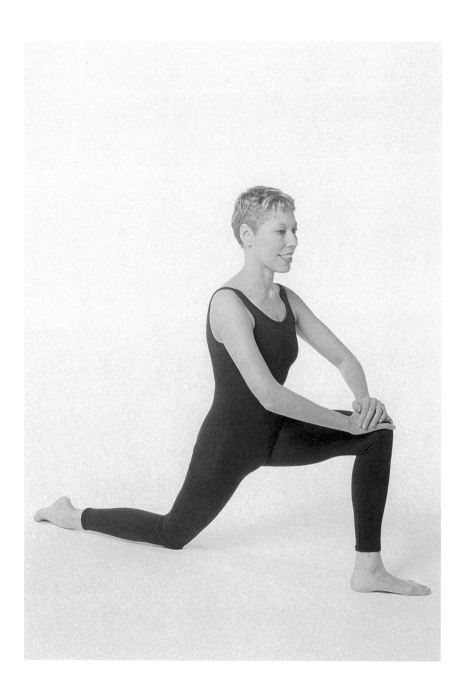

The Exercise Programme

33. Quadricep Stretch (advanced)

Assume the same position as in exercise 32, above. Holding your back foot, bend your knee and pull the foot towards your bottom. Keep your stomach in and don't arch your back. Hold for 30 seconds. Repeat four times, alternating legs.

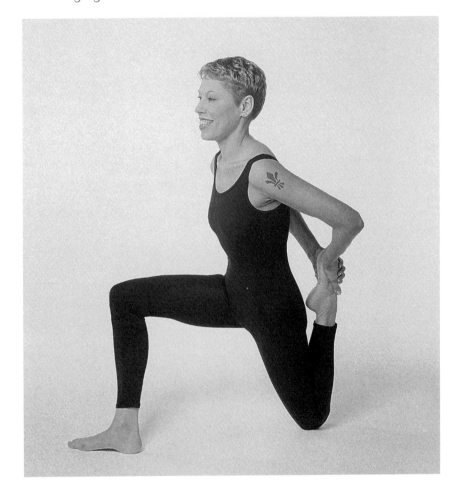

34. Lying Calf Stretch

Lying on your back, bend your knees into your chest. Place your hand behind the thigh of the leg that you're working, and stretch the leg towards the ceiling. Keep your foot flexed. Hold for 30 seconds. Repeat four times, alternating legs.

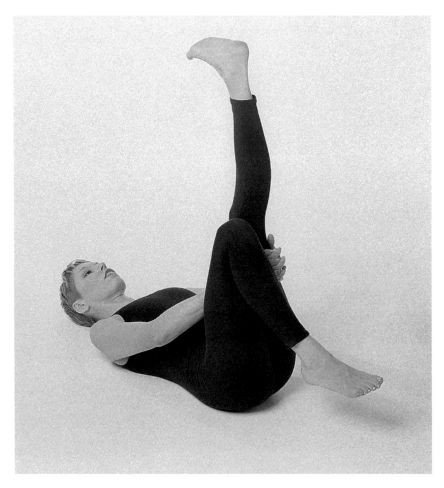

35. Standing Calf Stretch

Stand up straight. Take a step forward with your right leg and bend the knee slightly, and feel the stretch down through the back leg. Keep your heel down on the back leg. Do not bounce. Hold for 30 seconds. Repeat four times, alternating legs.

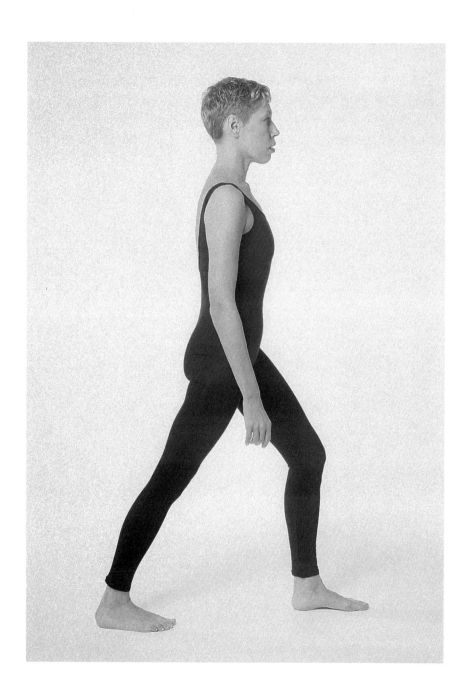

The Exercise Programme

36. Standing Hamstring Stretch

Place your foot (gently flexed) on a chair and extend your leg. Keep the standing leg slightly bent and your stomach in. Neck and shoulders are relaxed. Hips are level. Slide your hands down towards your foot. You should feel the stretch in the muscle between the knee and the hip. Hold for 30 seconds. Repeat four times, alternating legs.

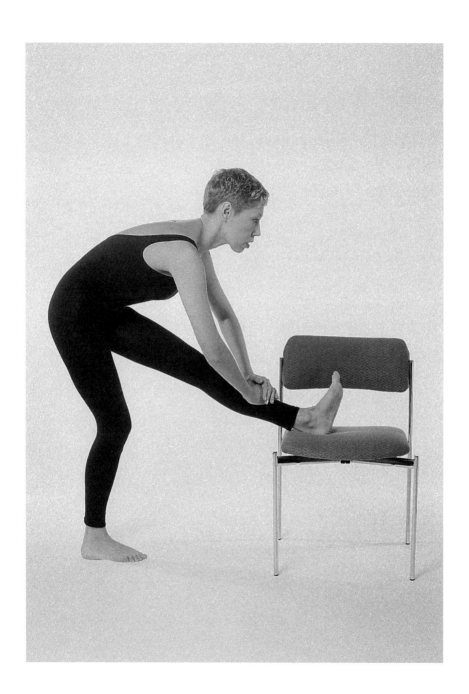

The Exercise Programme

37. Advanced Hamstring Stretch

Lie on the floor. Place a cushion under your head if this feels more comfortable. Pull your right knee in towards your chest. Place one hand behind your thigh, the other hand behind your calf. Gently stretch your right leg up towards your chest. Hold for 30 seconds. Repeat four times, alternating legs.

Watchpoints

- If your leg begins to shake – stop.

- If you feel any pain in your back during either of the hamstring exercises, relax. Your muscles may be too tight. Start with the first stretch only.

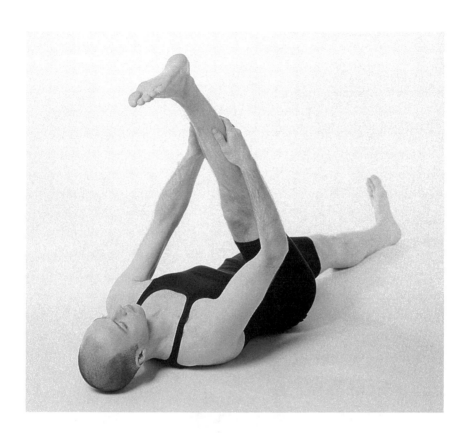

The Exercise Programme

38. Inner Thigh Stretch

Sit on the floor with the soles of your feet together, stomach in. Hold onto both ankles. Gently drop your chin to your chest, relax your shoulders and let your knees drop to the sides. Hold for 30 seconds. Repeat four times. If this is difficult, sit on a cushion to begin with.

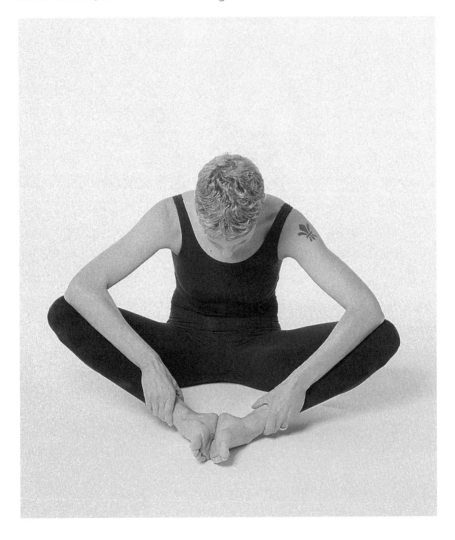

39. Advanced Inner Thigh Stretch

Lie on your back, with your legs up a wall. Let your legs fan out to the sides as far as is comfortable. Make sure your stomach is in, and your tailbone dropped. If you feel any pain in your knees, stop. Hold for 30 seconds. Bring your legs back together. Repeat four times.

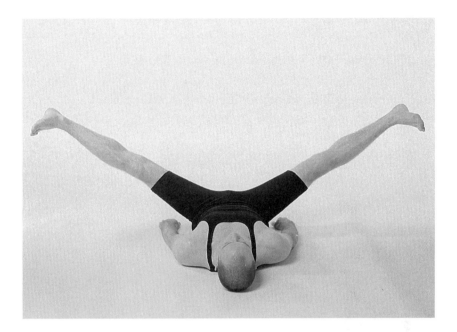

UPPER BODY EXERCISES

The following exercises will tone your arms, shoulders and chest. You can do second sets when your body builds up to it and follow them with the stretches.

One combination is press ups, dips and then repeat. An alternative would be a tricep press, bicep curl and then repeat.

The Exercise Programme

40. Press-up

To work your upper back, biceps and triceps

Get down on your knees and make a square with your body (as in the Cat Stretch, exercise 13). Place your hands slightly wider apart than your shoulders, palms flat with fingers facing in front of you. Gently tip your weight forwards, keeping your head in line. Keep your feet down. Breathe in as you bend your elbows and 'press' your head, shoulders and chest towards the floor. Breathe out as you raise yourself up again.

Keep your body in line and look at the same spot on the ground throughout. Do not arch your back and do keep your stomach in. Build up from 10 to 25 repetitions.

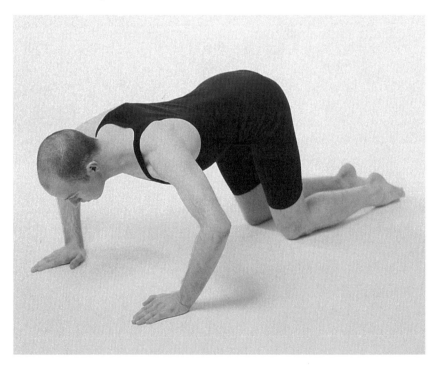

41. Press-up

To work upper back, biceps and triceps.

Start in exactly the same position as above. (All the same rules apply.) This time as you do the press-ups, cross your ankles and lift your feet off the ground. Don't do this if you have any pain in your knees. Build up from 10 to 25 repetitions.

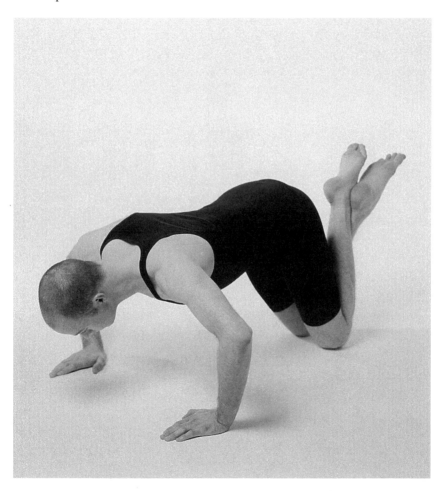

42. Tricep Dips

These will work your triceps and the backs of your arms.

....

Hold onto the edge of a chair in a sitting position, with your knees directly over your feet. Keep your hands facing forwards in line with your shoulders. Breathe in and slide down in front of the chair. Exhale and go back up, letting your arms do all the work (not your thighs). Do not raise your shoulders or lock your elbows, doing five or six, and gradually build up to 25 as you get stronger.

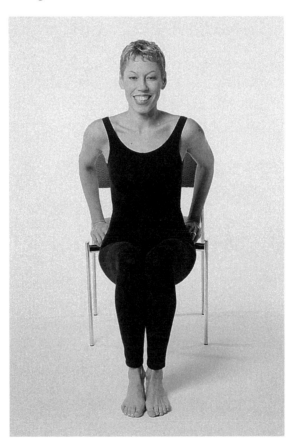

Use a two kilo hand weight for the following exercises.

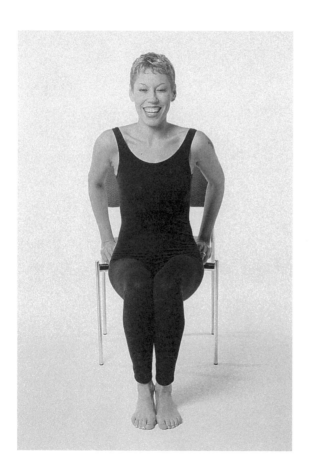

117

43. Tricep Press

Using a firm chair, make a square with your body. Place your left hand and knee on the chair, keeping your right leg straight on the ground. Keep your neck in line with the rest of your body. Holding the hand weight, lift your right arm up as high as you can keeping the elbow bent at a right angle, without twisting the body. Exhale as you straighten the arm behind you. Pause. Bend your arm back again. Repeat 10–15 times on each arm. You may do a second set.

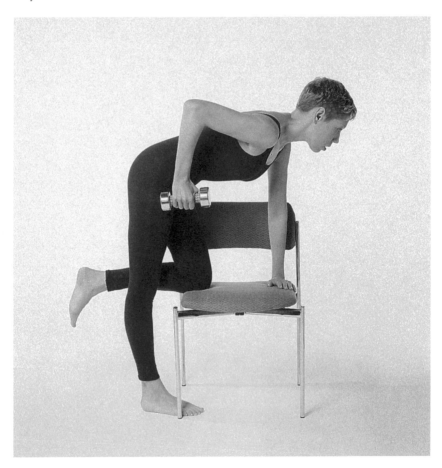

Watchpoint

Do not lock the supporting elbow, and keep your stomach in.

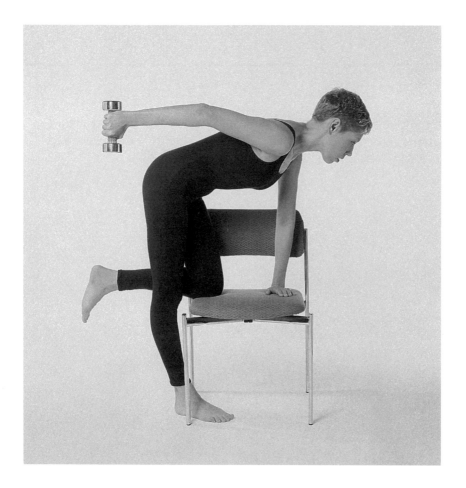

The Exercise Programme

44. Lat Exercise

Assume the same position as above. (All the same rules apply.) This time you're using your arm to pull up and down. As you 'pull' – feel your lats doing all the work – imagine you're pulling up weeds. Repeat as above.

Watchpoint

Do not use your shoulders to do the work in this exercise.

For the following exercises the same rules apply as for the initial 'perfect' posture exercise (see p.36).

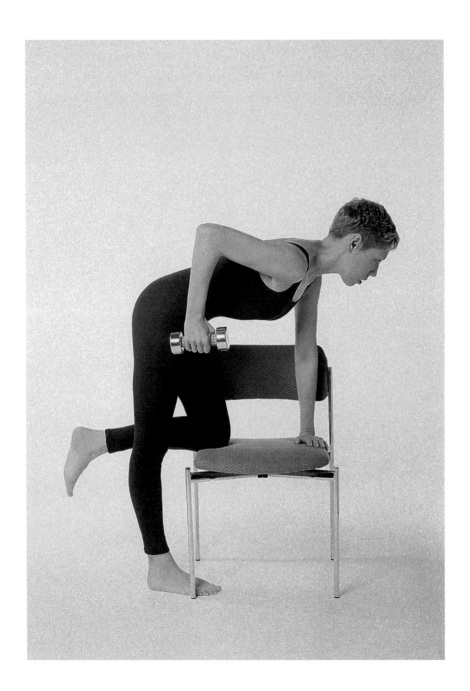

The Exercise Programme

45. Bicep Curl

Holding a two-kilo weight in each hand, breathe in and bend your arm up to shoulder level. Breathe out and straighten to waist level. Try not to rock as you do this. Repeat 10 to 15 times with alternate arms.

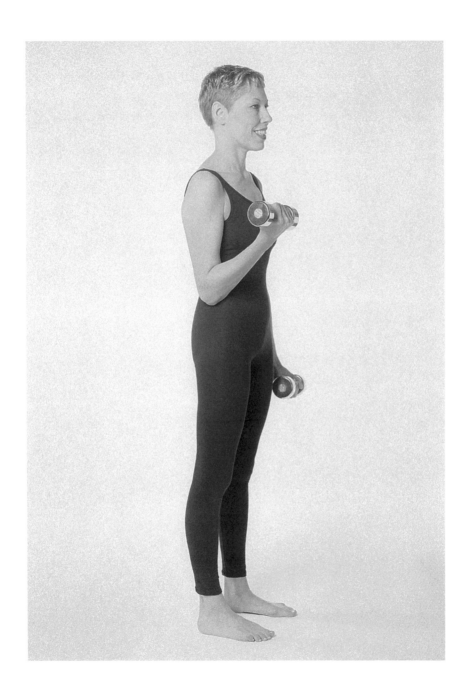

The Exercise Programme

46. Towel Stretch – for shoulders

Stand with your feet directly under your hips. Hold a rolled-up towel in front of you. As you exhale lift the towel up and over your head to touch your bottom, and reverse. Remember to keep your stomach and ribs in,

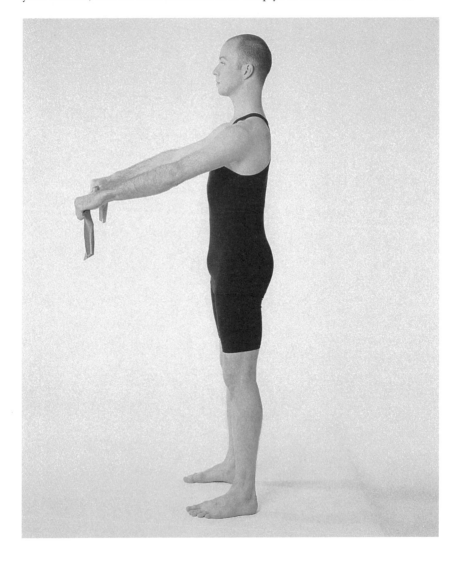

and not to arch your back. The longer the towel, the easier the stretch. Thus, as you become more flexible, you can shorten the towel. Repeat 10 times.

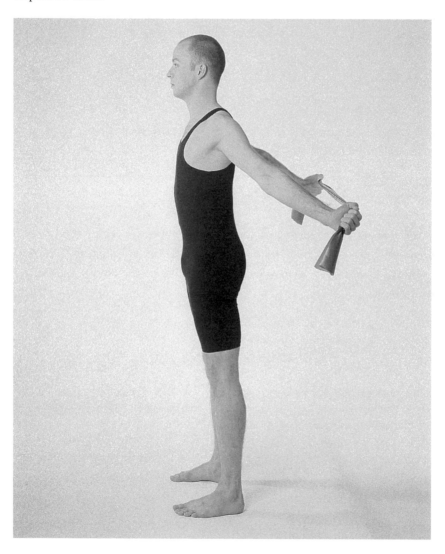

The Exercise Programme

47. Shoulder Stretch

This stretch can be done seated or standing. Cross one arm over the other and clasp your hands together. Gently push your elbows to the ceiling and feel your shoulders stretching. As you press your arms up, try and keep your shoulders down. Keep your elbows in line with your shoulders. Hold for 10 seconds and then relax. Repeat four times, alternating arms.

Watchpoint

If you feel any cramp or discomfort in your shoulders or arms, you are not yet flexible enough to do this.

The following arm exercises are done lying on your back. You should do them after your upper body work. They will help you to keep your shoulders flexible. Place a towel under your head if it feels more comfortable.

Watchpoint

In *all* of these exercises remember to keep your back in a neutral position: don't let your ribs lift. Keep your feet together, knees bent and thighs gently touching, with no tension in the lower back.

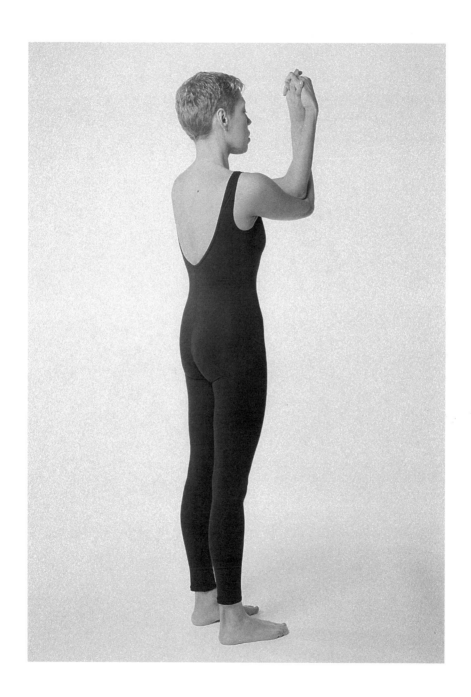

The Exercise Programme

48. Arms Opening

Lying on your back, raise your arms above your chest. Imagine you're a tulip, and as you breathe out, your arms gently open. As you breathe in, bring your arms back together. Keep the curve in the elbows. Repeat 10 times, opening and closing.

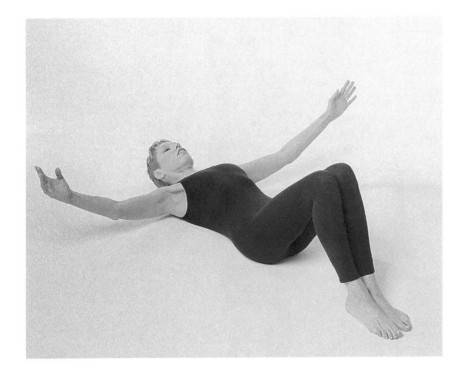

49. Backstroke

Start in the same position as above. Hold your arms over your chest. The palms face the wall in front of you. Keep your shoulders relaxed. As you breathe out, simultaneously one arm goes down in front of you and one behind you. Breathe in as you reverse the arms. Imagine you're doing the backstroke. Repeat 20 times, 10 on each side.

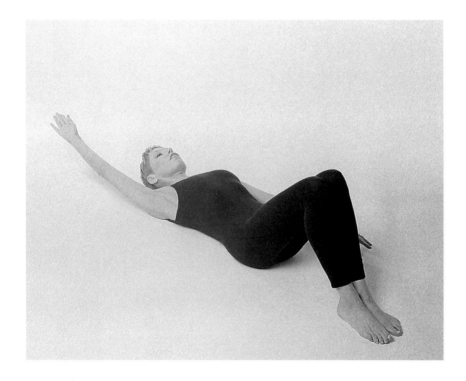

50. Shoulder Stretch

Assume the same position as in exercise 48 above. Place one hand gently over the other, so that you're making a diamond shape with your elbows. As you breathe out, take your arms as far back to the floor, past your ears, as you can without your back lifting. Repeat 10 times, alternating the hand on top.

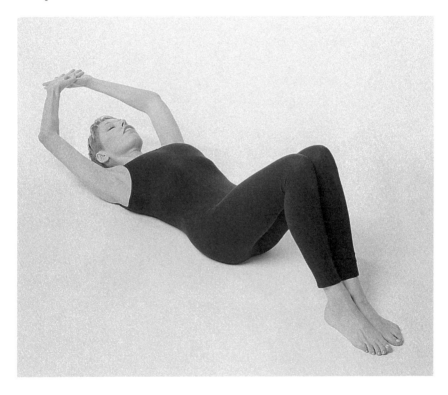

51. Arm Circles

Assume the same position as in exercise 48. With your arms stretched up above you, breathe out and make a circle, so that your hands touch the floor all the way behind you. Bring your arms back and stretch towards your hips. Repeat 10 circles one way and 10 going the other.

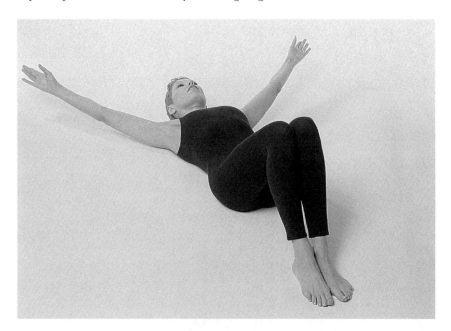

131

REMEDIAL EXERCISES

The following shoulder exercises can be done after upper body work. Although these are helpful for conditions such as scoliosis and repetitive strain injury (carpal tunnel syndrome), they are very gentle, relaxing exercises that can be done even if you do not suffer from any of these conditions.

The following three exercises can either be done on the floor, or sitting on a chair.

52. Single Shoulder Lifts

These work the shoulder joints and shoulder blades.

Make sure you are sitting comfortably. Breathe in, and slowly squeeze your right shoulder up to your right ear. Relax it down. Repeat with other shoulder. Do this to a count of four up, four down. Don't move your head. Repeat 10 times, alternating shoulders.

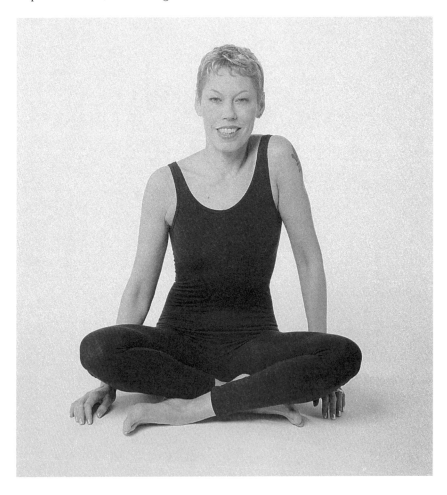

132

53. Double Shoulder Lifts

Sitting as above, squeeze both shoulders up to your ears. Make sure your hands are dangling loosely by your sides. If you feel you are arching your back, use a wall as support. Repeat 10 times.

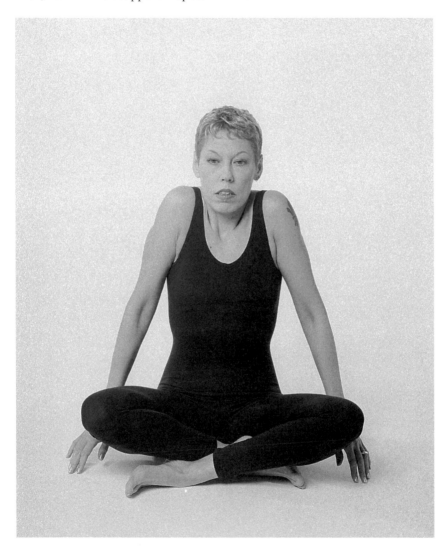

54. Shoulder Circles

Assume the same position as above. With both your hands on your shoulders, very gently circle both arms forward. Repeat 10 times. Then circle your arms backwards and again, repeat 10 times. If this feels uncomfortable, circle your shoulders with your arms at your sides.

The following exercises are for scoliosis.

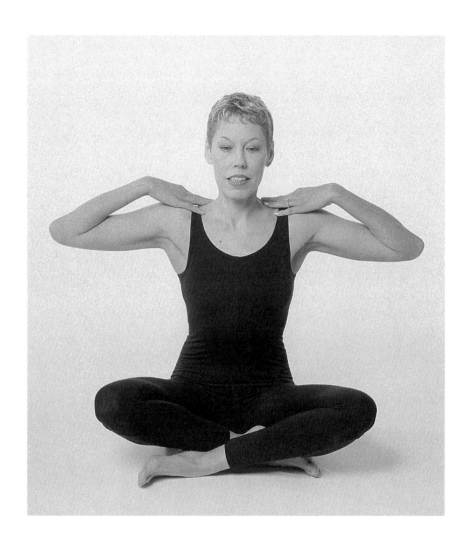

The Exercise Programme

55. Pelvic Tilt with One Leg Crossed

This is a basic pelvic tilt exercise (see exercise 1, p.44) – the only difference being that you cross one leg over the other.

Lie on your back, with your one leg crossed over the other. Arms should be relaxed at your sides, with palms facing the floor. Allow your back to keep its natural arch. Don't press it down – keep it in a neutral spine position. Try very hard not to tense your buttock muscles.

As you breathe out, gently tuck your pelvis under and curl your spine off the floor – through the lower back and into the middle back – until you're basically at the level just below your lower shoulder blades. Breathe in, keeping your neck long, and then very slowly roll down through the top of your spine, exhaling all the way down. Move one vertebra at a time, lowering yourself back onto the mat. Repeat 10 times, alternating legs.

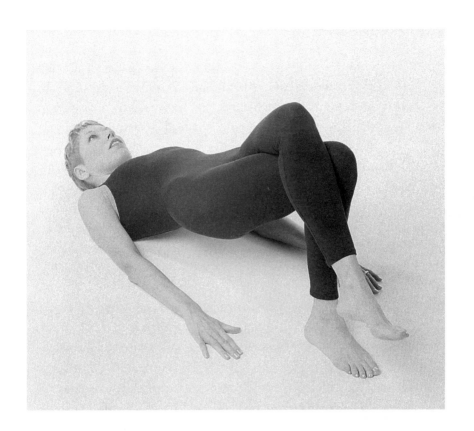

The Exercise Programme

56. One-arm Cat Stretch

This is exactly like the cat stretch in exercise 13 – the only difference is that one hand is on your back reaching towards the diagonal shoulder blade. If you've got scoliosis this may be difficult at first, and your hand may only go as far as your shoulder. You'll be able to stretch further as you get stronger.

Kneeling, make a square of the body. Keep your left hand under your left shoulder, fingers facing forwards. Place your other hand on your back and try to reach your diagonal shoulder blade. Knees should be hip-width apart. If your knees feel a little bit uncomfortable, just fold up a towel and put it under them. Place your feet gently on the floor and don't lock your elbow at any point during the stretch.

As you breathe out, drop your chin to your chest and curl your stomach into your spine. Press your upper back to the ceiling, trying not to rock back and forwards. As you breathe in, your tailbone lifts towards the ceiling, chest presses to the floor and your head gently lifts. Breathe in, and reverse the position. Relax your forehead to the floor. Relax your bottom onto your heels into the 'relaxation position' (see exercise 19, p.80), and just breathe. Repeat four times on each arm.

Watchpoints

- Don't lock your elbows.

- Don't lift your head too high or you may strain your neck.

- As you press your chest down to the floor in the reverse exercise, if you feel any pinching in your lower back you've gone too far.

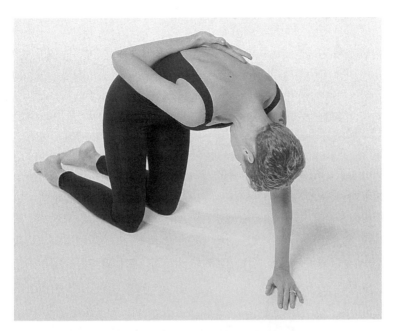

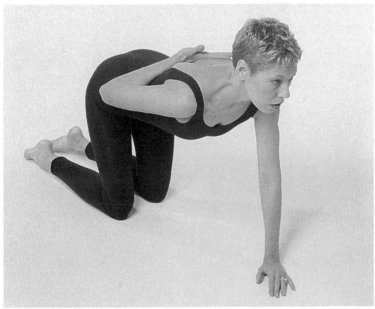

The Exercise Programme

57. Single Arm Stretch

Lie on your stomach and imagine you're a small starfish. Your arms are slightly wider than your shoulders, your forehead on the floor on a folded towel. Make sure your legs are comfortably apart and rotated slightly outwards. Place your right arm on your back reaching towards the left shoulder blade. Breathe out and let your left arm gently float off the ground. As your arm reaches away, think of your shoulder blade 'gliding'. You should feel this with the hand on your back. Make sure that as your stomach goes in, your pelvis drops. As you breathe out, don't grip your bottom.

Repeat four times, first on one side then the other. Then go into the relaxation position (see p. 80).

The following exercises are done against a wall. These will help to stretch out the shoulder blades and the upper back.

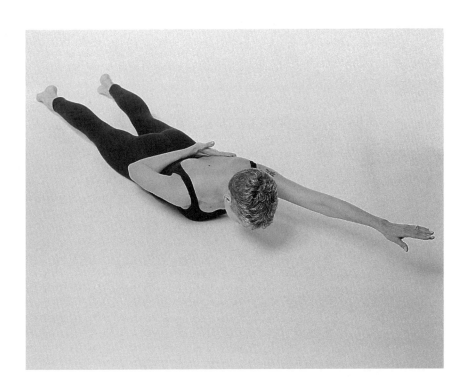

The Exercise Programme

58. Arm Stretch Against the Wall

Stand sideways on to a wall, about a foot away from it. Place your hand palm down on the wall. Do not arch your back. Very gently slide up the wall, leaning your body weight in to your palm, stretching your shoulder. Don't let the hips shift. Hold for a few seconds. Repeat four to six times, changing sides each time.

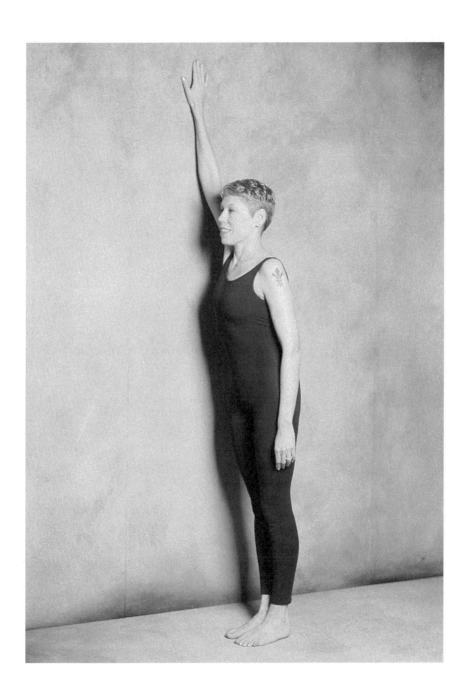

The Exercise Programme

59. Arm Stretch Against the Wall

Stand facing the wall, with one hand on top of the other against it. Keep your stomach in, tailbone dropped. Don't stick your bottom out. Gently stretch up the wall. Hold for a few seconds. Repeat 10 times, changing the hand on top.

The following two exercises are done kneeling on the floor. However, if you find this too difficult, you can sit on a chair and use a table to do them.

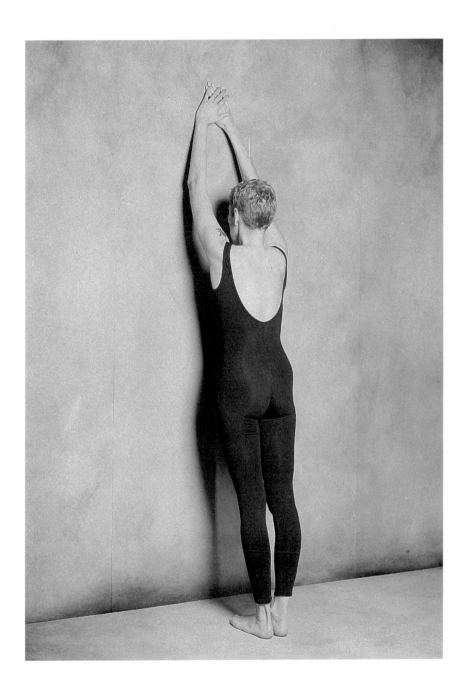

The Exercise Programme

60. Alternate Arm Lift

To work the shoulders and shoulder blades.

....

Sit down on your heels in the relaxation position (see exercise 19, p.80).
Have both hands wider than the shoulders and keep your head relaxed.
Slowly, without moving anything else, lift one hand off the floor. Hold for a
few seconds and relax back down. Don't twist your body or lift your head.
You should feel your shoulder doing all the work. Change hands and repeat
up to 10 times.

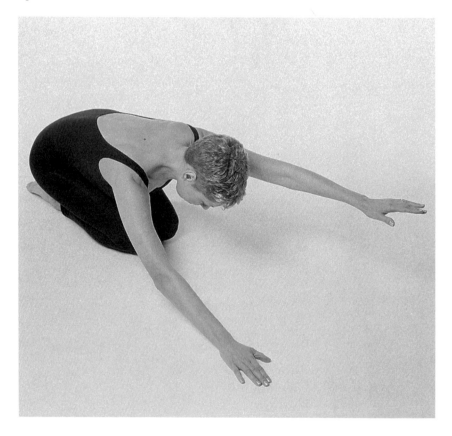

61. Alternate Arm Lift with Tennis Ball

Assume the same position as in exercise 60 above. This time, hold a tennis ball while lifting each hand.

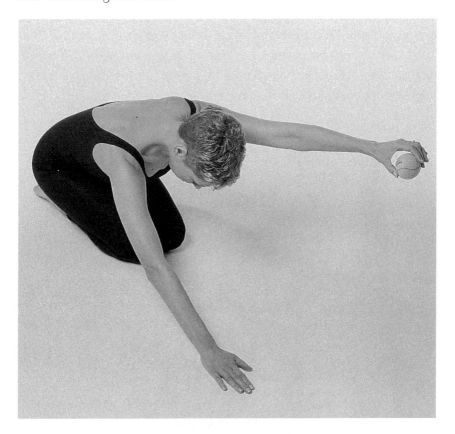

62. Basic Back of Hip and Buttock Stretch

Sit on the floor – you can lean against a wall. Stretch your left leg out in front of you. Cross your right foot over outside your left knee, keeping your right hand on the floor. Hold onto your right knee with your left hand, as you gently ease that knee into your chest. Then rotate your body round. The leg in front of you is parallel to the floor, keeping your toes to the ceiling and your shoulders down. Don't let your foot roll out of line to the knee. Feel the stretch through your buttock. Repeat four times, alternating legs.

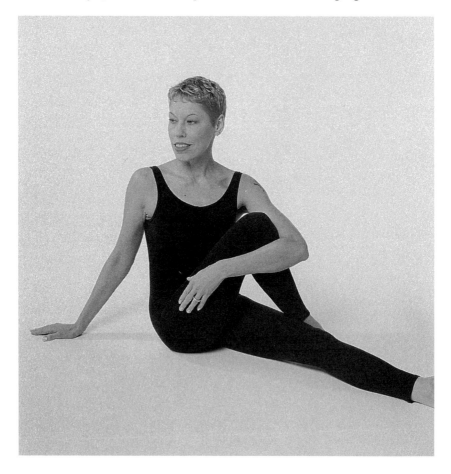

63. Basic Back Exercise

You should always do this exercise first if you've got a bad back.

Lie down on your stomach on the floor. Relax your head. Gently breathe in, and feel your stomach drop to the floor. Breathe out, pull your stomach into your spine, dropping your tailbone. Don't grip your bottom or tense your shoulders. Eventually, you will be able to get your fingers in between your stomach and the floor. Feel your stomach working. Repeat 10 times.

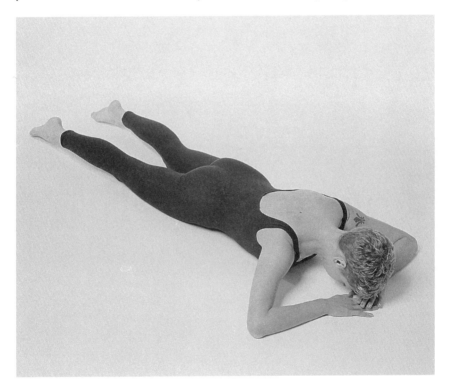

64. Ankle Circles

Lie down on your back, knees bent, with your hands holding behind your thighs. Gently circle your ankles 10 times one way and 10 times the other. Don't tense your toes.

The following four exercises are for repetitive strain injury (carpal tunnel syndrome). You can either kneel on the floor or sit on a chair.

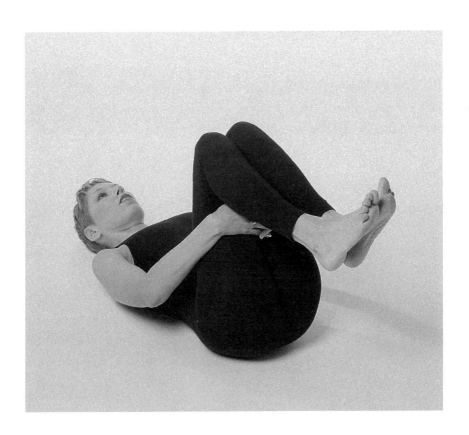

The Exercise Programme

65. Wrist Strengthening

Holding onto your wrist with the other hand, make a fist with your hand. The wrist is in neutral. Gently lower your wrist down *halfway* – and bring it back to neutral again. Think of this as a resistance exercise. Imagine you're resisting very slowly. You can also do this with your hand facing up. Repeat 10 times.

You can do this using a small weight too (e.g., a tin of beans), but not if you feel any pain.

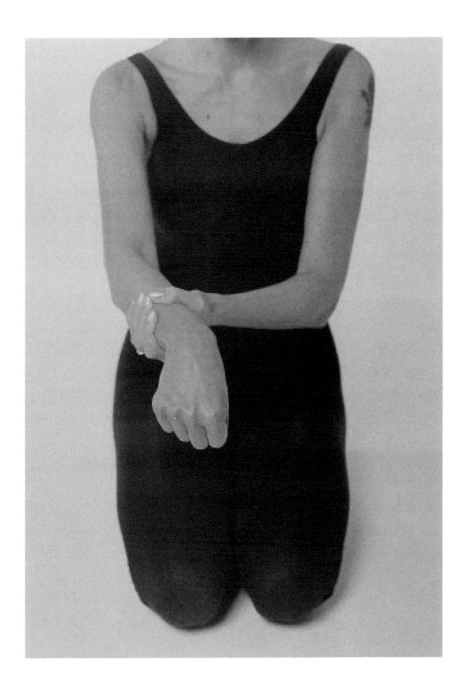

The Exercise Programme

66. Wrist Circles

Holding onto your wrist with the other hand, circle the wrist slowly one way, and then the other. Repeat 10 times, change hands.

Watchpoint

If you're doing these exercises correctly your hands and wrists will feel warmer.

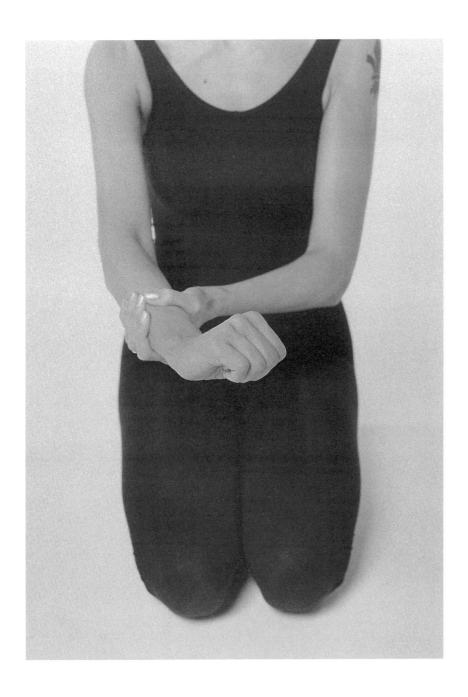

The Exercise Programme

67. Hand and Finger Stretch

Place your hands so that the tips of the fingers and thumbs are touching.
Imagine you're holding a soft ball. Press and resist your fingers – your
hands don't close. Keep your shoulders relaxed and hands level with
your chest.

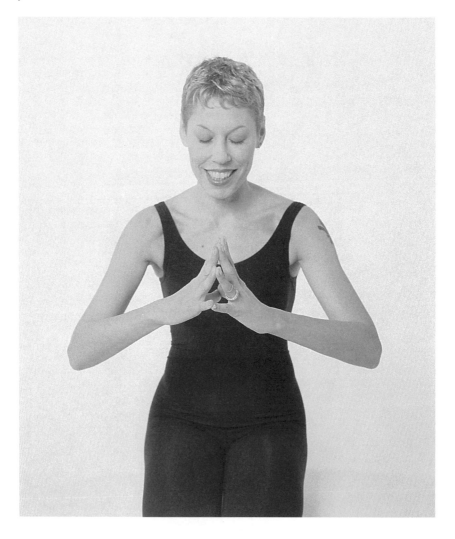

68. Wrist Stretch

Using a chair, place your hands on the seat, fingers towards you. Keep your elbows unlocked and gently lean your wrists into the chair. Don't press with your whole weight. Repeat four times. Shake your hands afterwards. Remember: don't lean too hard into the stretch.

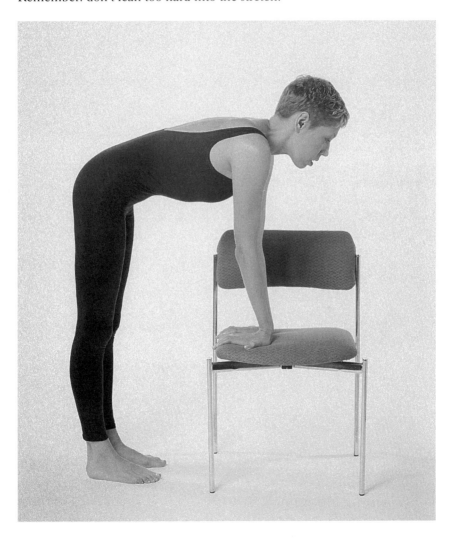

The Exercise Programme

69. Neck Stretch with Ball

This exercise will help to loosen up a tight neck.

Lying on your back, place a towel under your head and put a tennis ball under your chin. Very gently roll your head into your chest, lifting no higher than your shoulder blades. Then gently lower back down again. Repeat four times.

Watchpoints

- It's important that you do this exercise *only* four times – even if it seems as if you cannot feel a thing at the time.

- If you can feel any pain in your neck *do not do* this exercise.

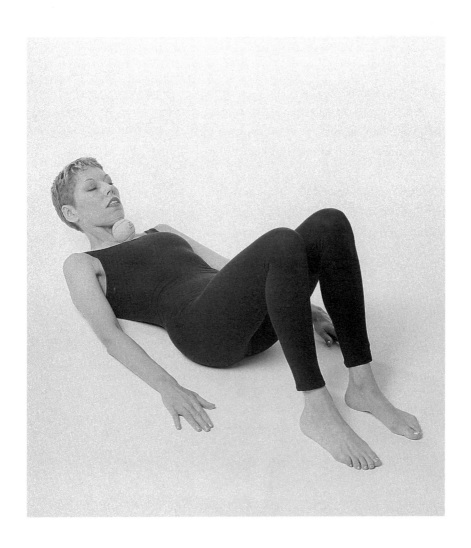

159

70. Rolling Up and Down the Wall

This is a great way to relax at the end of any programme, but if you have any back pain don't do this.

Lean your back against a wall. Remember to always keep the knees bent, otherwise you risk straining your back.

Breathe out, and very slowly drop your chin to your chest. It helps if you count as you do this. Start to roll your back down, as gently as you can. By the time you get to a count of eight, you want your shoulders to roll off the

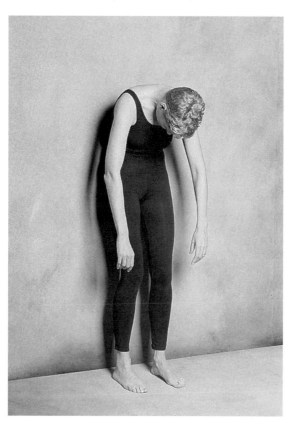

wall. If your legs start to shake, bend your knees a bit more. Roll down as far as you feel comfortable and count for 10–20 seconds. Your arms should now be hanging loosely by your side like a puppet's. Gently move your head from side to side. Pause, and try and roll up, very slowly. Repeat four times (twice down, twice up).

Watchpoint

If you've got low blood pressure don't do this, or you might feel faint.

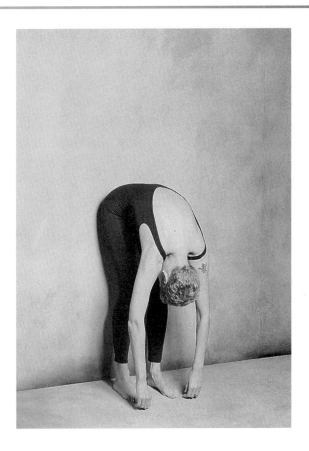

The Exercise Programme

6

Medical Remedial Work

For those of you who have repetitive strain injury (carpal tunnel syndrome), scoliosis or any other condition that affects muscles and joints, Pilates is a superb tool to use as you begin the journey towards helping and even reversing your condition. As previously stated, I absolutely believe *everyone* can and will improve, and even overcome, their physical difficulties with a safe and gentle group of exercises. You will be amazed at the body's ability to respond and rejuvenate, given the correct impetus. In Chapter 5 there are some specific exercises you can do every day to alleviate repetitive strain injury (carpal tunnel syndrome), scoliosis, sciatica or a bad back.

Note: The few remedial exercises contained in this book for each condition will not achieve the results possible in my studio and from individually taught programmes over an extended period of time.

REPETITIVE STRAIN INJURY (CARPAL TUNNEL SYNDROME)

This is a common problem amongst people whose work involves some kind of repetitive action, such as typing at a keyboard all day or playing a musical instrument. There are various types of injury which can be sustained in the muscles, tendons and ligaments in the hands and wrists from repetitive motions. The most common is the compression of the median nerve as it passes under the ligament that lies across the front of the wrist.

Symptoms appear after prolonged activity, and include tingling and weakness or numbness in the fingers and hands. Sufferers may also experience aching, burning or shooting pains in the wrists and hands, which frequently can spread to the forearms, neck, shoulders, upper back and upper arms. These symptoms get progressively worse until the person is barely able to use his or her hands at all, as the weakness makes it almost impossible to grasp objects properly. In the most severe cases the fingers may also swell up.

Conventional Treatment

Anti-inflammatory drugs, which may be prescribed to reduce the inflammation and swelling, aren't always effective. Painkillers can obviously help to relieve the pain, and wearing a splint can immobilize the wrist and alleviate discomfort.

Sufferers find that symptoms can come and go over the years. If the condition is not treated, the pain may become intolerable. Some people have to resort to surgery, which involves making an incision from the anterior of the wrist to the palm of the hand. The surgical effects are variable and symptoms may continue afterwards.

Body Maintentance Method

I have seen many people make a good recovery using the specific exercises I have evolved to treat this condition. These exercises are very gentle. They are designed to strengthen the hands and wrists and should be practised daily. As the hands and wrists get stronger and begin to regain proper mobility through exercise, the symptoms may disappear. Exercises 65, 66, 67 and 68 (see Chapter 5) are particularly recommended for this condition.

SCIATICA

Sciatica is a radiating pain along the distribution of the sciatic nerve, which affects the buttocks and backs of the legs. It frequently causes pain in the lower back, or lumbago. In severe cases it may spread to the calf of the leg. The most common cause of sciatica is from a prolapsed intervertebral disc. This causes pressure on one or more of the nerve roots which originate in the lower part of the spinal cord and make up the sciatic nerve. Sciatica may also occur for a number of other reasons. For example, this condition may happen suddenly when a person is lifting something heavy. The amount of pain varies, depending on which nerve roots are affected, and ranges from mild discomfort to acute pain.

Conventional Treatment

The first course of action is usually a few weeks of bed rest. Sometimes sufferers are prescribed a spinal support or corset. If there is no improvement, the next step may involve surgery in order to remove the compression of the disc on the nerve root.

Body Maintenance Method

Pilates-based exercises can do much to alleviate this debilitating condition. Exercises 14, 55, 56, 62 and 63 are particularly effective in gently strengthening the back.

SCOLIOSIS

Scoliosis is an extremely distressing condition that generates an S-shaped curvature of the spine. This is caused by a twist in the spine, which lead to the vertebrae becoming compressed and tilting to one side. In time this pressure can bring about fused vertebrae. Symptoms vary depending on the degree of the twist. There is generally a great deal of distress as the body struggles to accommodate this spinal imbalance, which forces the surrounding muscles into painful contortions.

Mild scoliosis may be barely noticeable, but in severe cases it leads to the formation of an unsightly hump and causes constant stooping, as the person is unable to stand upright. Scoliosis tends to first appear in adolescence and from then on, unless it is corrected while the body is still young and malleable, gets progressively worse.

Conventional Treatment

Treatment is usually very difficult. The most likely options for the scoliosis sufferer range from physiotherapy to surgical intervention. There are now several complex types of operations to try and correct it, or at least prevent the condition from worsening. However, these are not always successful.

Body Maintenance Method

I have devised a number of exercises designed to build up the weak muscles in the back and uncurl the spine, and have been witness to some remarkable changes.

Exercises 52–61 are particularly recommended.

Medical Remedial Work

BAD BACK

The back causes more problems than almost any other part of the body. The spinal column provides support to the entire body and is the centre of all movement. The muscles in the back link the vertebrae of the spine to each other. It is not surprising, then, that if these muscles are weak or damaged through injury, all sorts of problems affecting alignment and stability may occur.

Muscular pain and stiffness in the joints can transpire for many different reasons, for example congenital conditions, injury, weak muscles, a slipped disc, etc. The shock-absorbing discs betweeen the vertebrae may slip out of position and can damage the joints, leading to infections and degenerative problems. Pain varies depending on the cause of the problem and the person.

Conventional Treatment

Treatment may include anti-inflammatory drugs and painkillers, physiotherapy and surgery. Back problems can be notoriously difficult to eliminate.

Body Maintenance Method

Pilates-based exercises, as they focus on strengthening the muscles in the spine and abdomen, can be extremely beneficial for all sorts of back problems. See exercises 55, 56, 57, 63 and 64 in particular.

7

Case
Studies

GREG, 38

A combination of scoliosis and multiple sports injuries had left Greg, an insurance administrator, almost immobile.

'When I was younger, my life revolved around athletics. Growing up in Texas, I enjoyed all sorts of outdoor activities including tennis and horse-back riding. I also played American football for years. It was my ambition to become a professional football player. However, years of being thrashed around the pitch, breaking bones and sustaining various injuries really took their toll. Eventually, in my early twenties, I sustained a particularly nasty knee injury that forced me to abandon all athletic activities.

'It was recommended that I have surgery to repair the damage to the torn ligament. I ignored this advice. Subsequently, it was downhill all the way. As well as experiencing problems with my knees, all my old injuries came into focus. I discovered that I had scoliosis as well. My combination of ailments led to bouts of serious recurring back pain, aches and stiffness in my entire body, specifically in my elbows and arms. I couldn't bend or rotate my knees properly. I could barely do anything physical at all. In short – I was a wreck.

'After 10 years of distress a friend of mine suggested I try Pilates. I had already moved to London, and luckily I managed to stumble upon Lesley's Body Maintenance studio, which is only 10 minutes from my place of work. My initial impression was that the type of exercises Lesley suggested were far too simple to accomplish anything much. How wrong I was! After one or two sessions of going to Body Maintenance, I felt an improvement. Lesley showed me some simple stretches and mobility exercises. For the first time in years I could put my trousers on without having to use a coat hanger through the belt loops just to get them over my feet, which seemed like a major achievement. I quickly became a convert and started going to classes regularly – three times a week for one-and-a-half to two hours.

'Two-and-a-half years later, I feel physically fit. I rarely think about my back now and I've only had two incidents when it's played up – both caused by doing the wrong things. I get to travel a great deal and I used to worry about sitting in a plane and coping with the luggage. Now these considerations are no longer a major issue. All the pain has gone and I no longer feel that if I slip, sneeze or have to pick something up, my back is going to seize up.

'At present I can roller-blade, something I never thought I could do. I'm more sociable, as I'm not always worrying about hurting myself, I look better, my muscles are more defined and I've also managed to lose over 15 lbs in weight. Lesley's classes have totally changed my life on every level.'

JILL, 34

Hours of tapping on a keyboard led Jill, a tax advisor, to develop repetitive strain injury (carpal tunnel syndrome).

'About five years ago, I had to give up work because of repetitive strain injury (RSI). This condition was a direct result of my job, where I tapped away at the keyboard for about seven or eight hours a day. I think the problem worsened due to the fact that I had a computer that wasn't compatible to the rest of the network. There were always lots of system errors, which doubled my workload. This was very frustrating and I was in a state of extreme tension all the time.

'At first I had a few twinges in my hands, but after about nine months I started to get very sharp pains in my neck, numbness and shooting pains running up my fingers and into my wrists. Then it became sore elbows and shoulders. The pain was intolerable. At first I wasn't sure what was happening, then I was diagnosed with RSI. For six months I just hoped it would go away if I cut down on my keyboard work – but it didn't.

'I couldn't lead a normal life. I had no strength in my wrists and hands. I couldn't open doors, turn on taps, carry things, etc. Dressing was difficult and I could no longer drive. I couldn't bear people accidentally bumping into me or touching me. This was a big problem when I was travelling to work. To avoid any unnecessary pain I had to travel first class. After a year of this unfortunate situation, a friend of mine who also had RSI told me about Lesley. She'd been seeing her for about six weeks when she phoned to tell me how fantastic the classes were. So I decided to give it a try.

'Initially I went to classes twice a week, for an hour. Then I began going more often, usually about four times a week, and I did exercises at home. In the beginning Lesley had me doing some very gentle exercises. She was extremely clear on what I could and could not do. She had me do shoulder work, arm waving and holding small weights. I also did specific remedial exercises as well. For the first six weeks this was all quite painful and my hands and arms just felt limp. When everything became too painful I avoided all sorts of other activities. Lesley gave me the confidence to break this cycle. After six weeks I was no longer in pain. I felt slight discomfort as my arms and wrists began to get stronger. In the first six months the results were dramatic and I could almost return to normal life. I could drive again, open doors and do all the things I couldn't do before I met Lesley.

'Apart from the RSI, Pilates has also cured a 23-degree lumbar curve in my lower back, caused by scoliosis, which I never knew I had before I started Lesley's classes. Apparently, this may have been a contributory factor in my RSI.

'Although I can never go back to using a keyboard for more than 10 minutes a day, my life has vastly improved as a result of Lesley's classes. Compared to how I was five years ago, I feel amazing.'

BRENDA, 58

Double scoliosis had contorted Brenda's body to such an extent that she couldn't even stand up straight.

'For years I never knew what was wrong with me. I literally could not sit straight. My parents and teachers just thought I was lazy. As I aged a marked deterioration ensued. My posture was so dreadful that I started to develop a dowager's hump. I felt like an old crone.

'It wasn't until fairly recently that I discovered the reason for my appalling posture. In 1995 I was in a life-enhancement programme at the Canyon Ranch Spa in Arizona. They gave me a bone density test. This revealed that I had both lumbar and thoracic scoliosis – curves in my upper and lower back. The therapist did give me hope, however, and said that with the correct exercises the condition was reversible. Two weeks later, by marvellous coincidence, I was in London and happened to come across an article in a magazine recommending Lesley's Body Maintenance Programme. I phoned Lesley and she agreed to see me the following day. She made an immediate diagnosis and got me started on some very gentle exercises.

'I attended her classes every day. After six months the results were incredible. Slowly I was beginning to uncurve! A year later I returned to the Canyon Ranch. They could not believe the improvement. Of seven vertebrae stuck in my neck, only two now showed signs of fusion. I had also "grown" two inches and managed to lose 18 lbs in weight! The next time

I visited my couturier he was astounded. All my clothes had to be altered. He had to remake all the shoulders and hips because I was so much straighter.

'One might imagine that exercising for three hours every day could prove to be boring. On the contrary. I never know what to expect. When I hear "Brenda, you are floating," or "Levitate, you are oscillating," my body reacts even before I process the words. I straighten immediately – my body trusts Lesley unconditionally. Very often I arrive to see a glimmer in Lesley's eye and I know that a new and challenging exercise is on the way. When I am told that we are "winning" it is the highest form of compliment and spurs me on to strive all the more. Lesley is both teacher and fan – there is no end to the encouragement she offers.

'At present people comment how much better I look. Some even think I've had a face lift! Looking at old photographs I can see exactly what they mean. My previous stoop caused me to look as if I had no neck, and the muscles in my jaw were all pulled down and tense. This is no longer the case and my face no longer seems contorted.

'After three years, I feel like a different person. Apart from the dramatic physical results, I have changed both mentally and emotionally. Friends now tell me that I'm softer, calmer, more open and relaxed. I also feel more confident. Years of stooping had left me with very poor self-esteem. Now I'm much more assertive, outgoing and optimistic than I used to be. I truly believe that if you want something badly enough it can happen. Lesley has shown me that anything is possible.'

IAN, 67

A back injury sustained in his youth had left Ian, an actor, with an unrelenting legacy of pain.

'I've always led a very active life. When I was younger, I trained as a professional dancer. I then became an actor, so movement has always been an integral part of my life. Unfortunately, throughout most of my adulthood I had been plagued by back problems. The original problem started when I was 26. I'd sustained an injury to my back and had to be put in traction. Subsequently, I have had a history of going to osteopaths – a mixture of painkillers and osteopathy kept me going.

'The real crux came nine years ago when my partner of about 40 years became severely ill and I had to nurse him until he died. After that my back completely seized up – I couldn't turn my neck and became increasingly less mobile. I'd always enjoyed gardening and walking and now I could no longer do either of these things at all. My physiotherapist at the time suggested I see Lesley. I had some knowledge of Pilates, as I'd done it before. However, that was when I was much healthier, and the classes I took were very much state-of-the-art type affairs. Lesley's Body Maintenance techniques are very different. She also completely understands injury.

'My first impression of Lesley was that she had an extraordinarily innate sense of caring. She intuitively seems to understand a person's needs. She's very aware that people in pain are terribly afraid of moving. Lesley treats the source of the problem by dealing with all the peripherals. She taught me how it was possible to very gently and safely work through the pain, so that I could start re-building my weak muscles.

'Lesley started me off on an extremely gentle programme, twice a week. Very gradually this was increased to four times a week. The results have

Case Studies

been quite amazing. After only eight weeks, she'd "cured" my upper back problems. Over the last few years the difference in my strength and mobility has been enormous. After about a year virtually all my pain had gone. I was able to throw away my painkillers. Now, I only get the odd twinge and that's when I've been sitting in one position for too long. My physiotherapist is totally amazed at how I've managed to build up so much muscle on my back. I can even touch my toes! Thanks to Lesley I'm now about ten times as supple as someone else of my age. I also feel very fit. Lesley's unique approach has given me a completely new lease of life. Instead of dreading getting older, I'm now more active and fulfilled than I could ever have hoped to be before.'

JASMINE, 23

Jasmine, a successful model, had returned to work from a six-month sabbatical and was dismayed that she no longer recognized her body.

'I had always taken very good care of myself. I have been modelling since the age of 17 and always maintained the same dress size and weight. Models are scrupulous when it comes to body image. I am a very tall woman and that too is a great asset as I always appear to be long and lean. While most people think the life of a model is all glamour, nothing could be further from the truth. Early morning shoots, constant travel and the rush during the seasonal fashion collections gave me very little time for myself. When my brother suggested a joint business venture, I jumped at the chance to have something to connect to when I stopped modelling.

'Six months down the line I returned to my agency to resume my former life and was appalled at the reception I received. From my posture to the distribution of body weight it was clear that something was drastically wrong. My agent suggested that I visit Lesley Ackland's Body Maintenance Studio to get back into shape.

'I was unprepared for the calm, no-nonsense kindness Lesley offered. After a detailed discussion, down to my earliest biology/biography, many issues came to light.

'Yes, I was tall, but had I always enjoyed my "stature"? Recalling very painful experiences, from being teased at school to always feeling awkward when meeting men (my first consideration was height rather than character), I began to understand what had occurred. Lesley explained that my model's fashionable "slouch" had far preceded my career. It had begun when I was about 13 years old, and after 10 years my posture was dreadful. Other problems stemming from my poor alignment were slack stomach muscles and backaches. During my break I had done cursory exercises – sit-ups and jogging – but these did not keep my body toned.

'Lesley gave me postural exercises and explained how her routine, if adhered to, could correct my posture and re-distribute my weight through tightening and toning areas of my body. I was amazed at the type of programme I was given. I had imagined an endless repetition of boring, punishing exercises, i.e., no pain – no gain. The exercises were excellent and left me with a feeling of accomplishment and well-being. I faithfully attended Lesley's Body Maintenance classes three times a week. I not only achieved the shape I wanted, but received an unexpected gift as well. I underwent a metamorphosis. Lesley gave my body a new vocabulary – lissome, lithe, supple. I have a new image of myself, one which I truly like and appreciate.

'In a way I am grateful for the problem which brought me to Lesley – an old wound has been addressed and I have never looked or felt better. I keep myself "maintained" at Lesley's studio, and, when on a shoot or assignment,

Case Studies

I have the ability to do my exercises whenever and wherever I wish. I am simply delighted.'

8

Conclusion

The benefits of embarking on this exercise programme are manifold. As in any DIY book, until you familiarize yourself with all the material and go through it at your own pace, it may seem a bit confusing. You will find that once you co-ordinate your movements with the correct breathing any apprehension will soon vanish.

While the material is still fresh, before you close this book, why not try some of the simple visualization exercises right now? Close your eyes – scan your body – visit each area. What do you feel? Is any area painful or weak? Do you immediately focus on one area? Try some of the simple postural exercises to get a feeling of alignment. Imagine how you wish to appear.

Your body represents the sum of its parts – therefore each part must be fully conversant with the others. Fluency can be achieved by allowing the mind–body–spirit connection to evolve. This is a challenge which can be met with calm determination and a vision of purpose. You now have the tools. Good luck!